W9-CDA-834

LIVE
YOUNGER
LONGER

INSIGHTS FROM A MAYO CLINIC CARDIOLOGIST AND CANCER SURVIVOR

Stephen Kopecky, M.D.

MAYO CLINIC PRESS

Medical illustrations and photo credits

All photographs and illustrations are copyright of MFMER except for the following:
NAME: shutterstock_768496726 PAGE: 10-11 CREDIT: © SHUTTERSTOCK / NAME: 1994ChestXrayLungMet PAGE: 14 CREDIT: © Dr. Stephen L. Kopecky / NAME: 1994April PAGE: 15 CREDIT: © Dr. Stephen L. Kopecky / NAME: 2017Ceremony PAGE: 15 CREDIT: © Dr. Stephen L. Kopecky / NAME: 1999Christmas PAGE: 19 CREDIT: © Dr. Stephen L. Kopecky / NAME: IMG_3251 PAGE: 51 CREDIT: © Andy Fickman / NAME: 2016ChristmasPatagonia PAGE: 67 CREDIT: © Dr. Stephen L. Kopecky / NAME: shutterstock_1912135909 PAGE: 68 CREDIT: © SHUTTERSTOCK / NAME: shutterstock_750448753 PAGE: 92-93 CREDIT: © SHUTTERSTOCK / NAME: shutterstock_1288402915 PAGE: 100 CREDIT: © SHUTTERSTOCK / NAME: EmilyAtDX PAGE: 150 CREDIT: © Dr. Stephen L. Kopecky / NAME: EmilyPreDX PAGE: 150 CREDIT: © Dr. Stephen L. Kopecky / NAME: EmilyPostDX PAGE: 150 CREDIT: © Dr. Stephen L. Kopecky / NAME: SLK_Office PAGE: 154 CREDIT: © Dr. Stephen L. Kopecky / NAME: 1985WeddingSLKandLFK PAGE: 160 CREDIT: © Dr. Stephen L. Kopecky / NAME: shutterstock_1069235309 PAGE: 194-195 CREDIT: © SHUTTERSTOCK / NAME: shutterstock_78101914 PAGE: 207 CREDIT: © SHUTTERSTOCK / NAME: shutterstock_154387970 PAGE: 207 CREDIT: © SHUTTERSTOCK / NAME: shutterstock_218815381 PAGE: 207 CREDIT: © SHUTTERSTOCK / NAME: shutterstock_251894638 PAGE: 207 CREDIT: © SHUTTERSTOCK / NAME: shutterstock_1493262659 PAGE: 207 CREDIT: © SHUTTERSTOCK

Published by Mayo Clinic Press

© 2021 Mayo Foundation for Medical Education and Research (MFMER)

MAYO, MAYO CLINIC and the Mayo triple-shield logo are marks of Mayo Foundation for Medical Education and Research. All rights reserved. No part of this book may be reproduced, stored in a retrieval system, or transmitted, in any form or by any means, electronic, mechanical, photocopying, recording or otherwise, without the prior written permission of the publisher.

This book is intended only as an informative guide for those wishing to learn more about health issues. It is not intended to replace, countermand or conflict with advice given to you by your own physician. The ultimate decision concerning your care should be made between you and your doctor. Information in this book is offered with no guarantees. The author and publisher disclaim all liability in connection with the use of this book.

The views expressed in this book are the author's personal views, and do not necessarily reflect the policy or position of Mayo Clinic.

For bulk sales to employers, member groups and health-related companies, contact Mayo Clinic, 200 First St. SW, Rochester, MN 55905 or SpecialSales-MayoBooks@mayo.edu.

ISBN 978-1-893005-67-9
Library of Congress Control Number: 2021937321

Printed in the United States of America

To my wonderful wife of the past 35 years, Linda.

You are the oxygen that I breathe.

From the author

On my 40th birthday, having just gone through extensive cancer treatment, my oncologist told me that the CT scan looking for residual cancer showed a lump in my abdomen requiring further surgery. That was the second cancer in my life and, unlike the first cancer which occurred when I was in medical school and for which I underwent surgery and radiation therapy, this cancer had been treated with surgery and months of chemotherapy.

Fighting this cancer had been the focus of my existence. I had come to appreciate the proverb, "A healthy person has a thousand wishes, a sick person only one." At that point I decided that if I was fortunate enough to recover and survive, I needed to do all I could to make sure I never had cancer again. This led me to try to learn things I could do to prevent future cancer and major illness.

At the time I was an invasive cardiologist treating heart attacks and doing coronary angioplasties, which meant that my daily work was on the treating side, not the prevention side, of medicine. Learning how to prevent disease was somewhat new to me. What I learned surprised me. I found out that although I had two prior cancers, heart disease was the most likely future cause of me passing from this earth. I also discovered that six key lifestyle habits lead to heart disease and are also the major causes of other plagues in our current world: cancer, Alzheimer's disease, diabetes and likely many more.

Finally, I had to come to grips with a subject most 40-year-olds don't want to face, which was my eventual and inevitable death. Looking into this further, I found that there are basically four patterns of health, or lack thereof, toward the end of life: sudden death within an hour, rapid death over a few months, long-term frailty before death and organ failure. The latter two usually mean years, if not decades, of illness.

So, six daily habits lead to multiple chronic diseases that result in four patterns of illness during a lifetime. Getting back to the proverb, I realized that if I was fortunate enough to fully recover from this second cancer, I wanted to have the best health that I could, for as long as I could, for the rest of my life. In other words, I wanted to live younger longer. This ultimately led me to the prevention side of medicine, which is what I do now every day. I wrote this book to help others. It summarizes what I have learned about what we can all do to *Live Younger Longer*.

Stephen Kopecky, M.D.

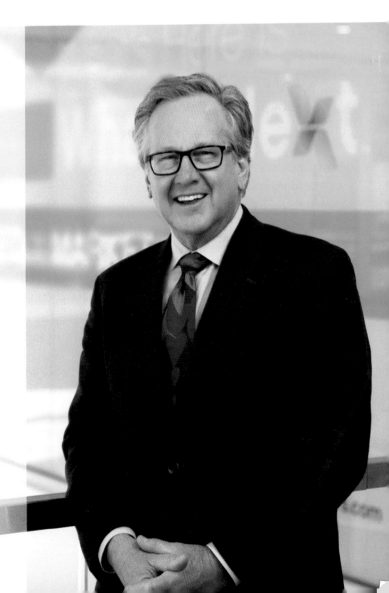

Stephen (Steve) Kopecky, M.D., is a cardiologist at Mayo Clinic, Rochester, Minn. He specializes in helping people lower their risk of heart disease and of having a heart attack or stroke. He also helps individuals with heart disease reduce their risk of further complications.

Acknowledgments

I am indebted to Mayo Clinic for allowing me to write this book and for their deep support throughout the process. I also want to extend my sincere gratitude to the many people who helped this book become a reality:

To the Mayo Clinic Press team including Dan Harke, Karen Wallevand, Amanda Knapp, Jennifer Koski, Heather LaBruna, Allison Vandenberg-Daves, Laura Waxman and Jodi Wentz for their talented help. To Rachel Haring Bartony, my editor, who spent countless hours teaching me the essentials of writing and organizing a book, and for her many excellent ideas and insights.

To my colleagues — doctors, nurse practitioners, nurses, dietitians and exercise physiologists who work in the Cardiovascular Health Clinic of Mayo Clinic, Rochester, Minn. — for continuing to teach me about the best way to prevent disease.

To Dr. Bruce Johnson, Dr. Ray Squires and Dr. Tom Allison for educating me from their vast wisdom about the exercise physiology of the human body.

To Dr. Amit Sood and Dr. Edward Creagan, two past colleagues from Mayo Clinic who have given me valuable advice on the mindset necessary to write a book and on how to communicate with patients and readers.

To my mentors, Dr. Robert Frye, Dr. Gerald Gau and Dr. George Gura, all wonderful humanitarians who showed me how to communicate with patients.

To Tom Root and Dr. Ming-Kai Chin of The Foundation for Global Community Health for showing me that reaching the world's children is the best way to prevent future disease.

To my father, Dr. Leon Kopecky, and my mother, Dr. Ina Moodie Calhoun Kopecky, from whom I learned that physicians are required to not only cure an illness, but also heal a patient.

To my wife, Linda, who's always given me unconditional love and support, and my children and children-in-law, Emily and Tim Miller and Dr. Katy Kopecky and Dr. Ben Kopecky, who have helped me tremendously with this book by giving me insights from the millennial generation about what's important in life.

Finally, to all my patients who I have been fortunate enough to know — they have taught me so much about their illnesses and the causes through their honest discussions.

Contents

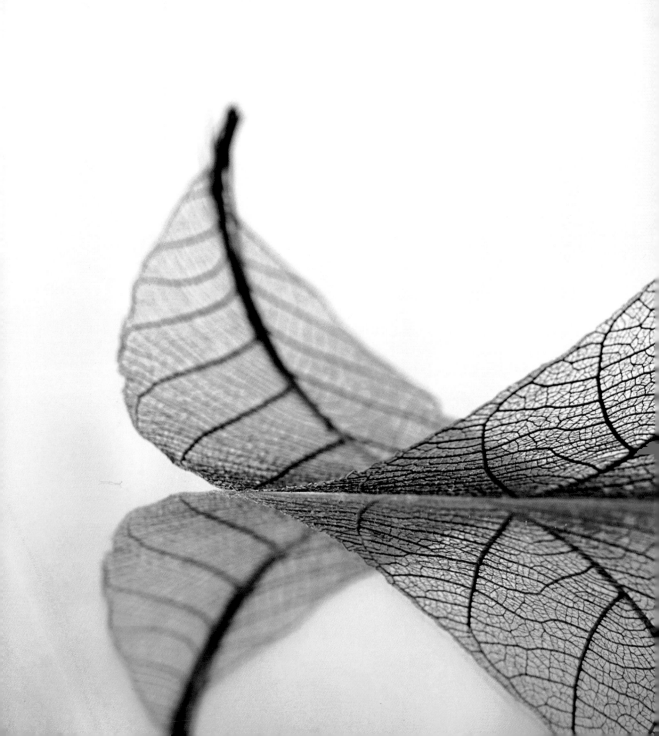

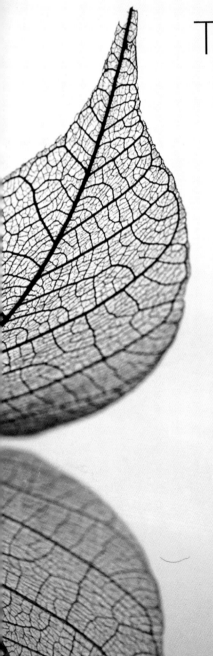

PART 1

The state of our health

"DEATH IN OLD AGE IS INEVITABLE, BUT DEATH BEFORE OLD AGE IS NOT."

— British research pioneer Sir Richard Doll

CHAPTER 1

What kills us

I always knew I was going to be a heart doctor like my father. I had it all planned out: One day I'd return to my hometown of San Antonio and join him in his practice, working side by side to improve the health of the community I grew up in. That was the plan anyway. But sometimes life takes you on a different course, opening your eyes to other possibilities and leading you to new places.

MY STORY

In the early 1980s, I was a 20-something who had the world by the tail. In my fourth year of medical school at the University of Texas in Houston, I was ready to travel the country, doing monthlong rotations at different medical institutions. This process, common for medical students in their final year, was going to help me figure out where

I eventually would want to train. I had an amazing first month in Rochester, Minnesota, at Mayo Clinic, then moved on to the University of California, Los Angeles.

A few days after arriving in LA, I felt a testicular lump. The lump was hard and painless — red flags of a cancerous growth. A biopsy confirmed that I had a form of testicular cancer called seminoma. Testicular cancer is one of the top five causes of death in young men. Fortunately, in my case, my cancer didn't appear to have spread, which greatly increased my chance of survival.

I returned to Houston for treatment, undergoing six weeks of radiation at MD Anderson Cancer Center. As any cancer patient will tell you, treatment weeks can feel more like months. Those six weeks did indeed feel like six months. As a side effect of my radiation therapy, I was sleeping 16 hours a day. The days and nights went by in a blur.

But I was young and looked at the whole episode as a bump in the road, something that wouldn't affect me much over the long run. I was ready to put it all behind me and forge ahead with my career in medicine.

My primary doctor at the time said he felt that my experience with cancer would change my career path — maybe even make me want to go into a cancer treatment field. But I thought to myself, there's no chance this will deter me from my cardiology goal.

I ended up spending three years training in internal medicine at Mayo Clinic and stayed there to complete cardiology training. I realized how fortunate I was to spend that early month at Mayo Clinic as a fourth-year medical student before my cancer was found. If I had planned on visiting Mayo Clinic even a month later, I'm sure I wouldn't have made that visit.

My time at Mayo Clinic was life changing. Watching medical teams work together to do everything in their power to help patients — I felt like few institutions did it as well as Mayo Clinic did. And after being a cancer patient, that was something I could appreciate.

During this time I also married my wife, Linda, and we had our first child, Emily. Once training was complete, our little family left for Texas to fulfill my dream of prac-

ticing with my father. But the pull of Mayo Clinic remained. Two years after returning to San Antonio, we were on our way back to Mayo Clinic, where I took a position as a cardiologist. Our family eventually grew to three children and life was good.

When I was 39, I found another lump, which turned out to be testicular cancer again. But this time was very different. This was a more aggressive form called embryonal carcinoma, and it had spread to my lungs and other parts of my body. Treatment would be more grueling — six months of chemotherapy and surgery to remove any residual cancer.

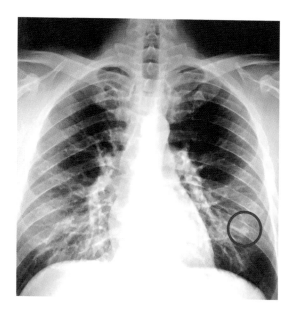

A chest X-ray in 1994 revealed the spread of embryonal carcinoma to my lungs (circled). I keep this photo by my desk to remind me of how fortunate I am to be here.

Following treatment, I was, for the second time, considered cured. It was at this point that I had a realization: I had had cancer twice before the age of 40. I had a family history of cancer. I also had a wife and three young children. Early death was not an option in my mind. I needed to do everything I could to prevent this from happening again.

The thought of recurrence is one that never really leaves a cancer survivor. And it's understandable to think that ultimately it may be what kills you. That was my thinking initially. But as a cardiologist, I saw another stark reality. As I looked at the growing number of cardiovascular disease-related deaths worldwide, I realized that, statistically, heart disease was also a foe — a foe that in many cases was more likely than cancer to kill a cancer survivor.

THE BIG SHIFT

Today, heart disease is the No. 1 cause of death in the world, causing close to a third of all deaths worldwide. But this wasn't always the case.

Over a century ago, a person's greatest health threats came from infectious diseases. These diseases spread from person to person, often through contaminated water, inadequate hygiene or airborne transmission. The top causes of U.S. deaths in the early 20th century were influenza, pneumonia, tuberculosis (sometimes referred to as "consumption") and gastrointestinal infections.

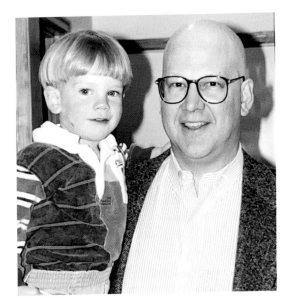

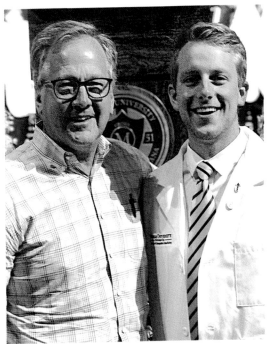

My son, Ben, was 2 (top) in 1994 when I received chemotherapy. In 2017 (bottom), I was privileged to attend his white coat ceremony when he began medical school.

Vaccines weren't available yet, poor hygiene and inadequate sanitation were rampant, and knowledge of how to prevent or treat these diseases was limited. It was the perfect storm for the spread of potentially fatal illnesses. Heart disease also made the top 10 causes of U.S. deaths in 1900. But this was mostly heart disease stemming from infections or valve problems.

Looking at the chart on the right, you can see the shift in the top causes of death in the U.S. over the course of the 20th century, even as the population grew exponentially. Influenza and pneumonia are no longer at the top. Heart disease — the kind that damages the heart and blood vessels and that's primarily due to unhealthy lifestyle factors — now occupies the top spot by a substantial margin. Chronic noncontagious (noncommunicable) diseases are much more likely than infectious diseases to kill us now.

Perhaps what's most troubling is that the majority of these deaths are, to some degree, preventable. We know that lifestyle measures such as eating a healthy diet, avoiding tobacco and staying active can help prevent many of today's leading causes of death.

LIVING THE MODERN LIFE

So, what happened over the years to create this shift? The chart on the right illustrates an important concept. What keeps us healthy or makes us sick evolves as the environment around us and social conditions of a society change.

In the last century, medical advances such as vaccinations, antibiotics, improved public health systems and better health education lessened the impact of contagious diseases. At the same time, new behaviors — such as more people smoking cigarettes and driving automobiles — meant a greater number of deaths from causes such as lung cancer and car accidents.

Advances in technology and testing helped to uncover previously unknown diseases and better treat existing ones. On the other hand, advances in manufacturing and industry greatly influenced our daily activities, our diets and, ultimately, our health.

Instead of walking to the store, most of us drive there. Instead of a job that entails manual labor or physical exertion, a great number of us spend most of our workdays seated in front of computers. Some people have jobs that require working at night, altering their sleeping and eating patterns.

Our ancestors used to rely on plants they foraged and wild animals they hunted. The introduction of farming and manufacturing practices has made it much easier to access food. And as a result, our diets have shifted to include more dairy, cereal, refined sugars, refined vegetable oils, salt and fatty meat.

Modern processed foods, while convenient and inexpensive, have lost many of the healthy qualities of whole, unprocessed foods. In 1970, only 0.2% of the sugar we consumed was from high-fructose corn syrup. By 2000, this processed sweetener made up

LEADING CAUSES OF DEATH IN THE LAST CENTURY

UNITED STATES, 1900, 1950 AND 2000

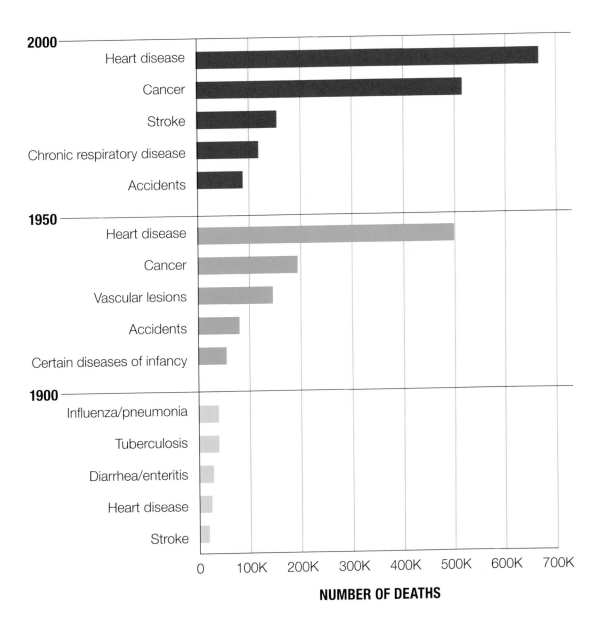

NUMBER OF DEATHS

Based on Centers for Disease Control and Prevention

HABITS DRIVE MODERN DEATHS

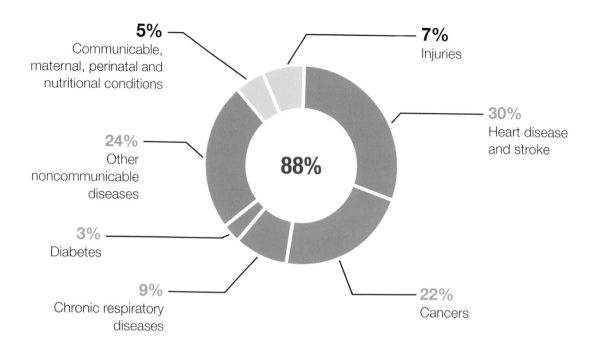

5%
Communicable,
maternal, perinatal and
nutritional conditions

7%
Injuries

30%
Heart disease
and stroke

24%
Other
noncommunicable
diseases

88%

3%
Diabetes

9%
Chronic respiratory
diseases

22%
Cancers

The vast majority of deaths in the U.S. are caused by noncontagious (noncommunicable) diseases such as heart disease and stroke, cancers, lung diseases, diabetes, and others. Most of these diseases are driven by unhealthy lifestyle habits.

Based on Centers for Disease Control and Prevention, World Health Organization

almost a third of our diet's sugar content. And the same goes for fats. In the 20th century, our use of vegetable oils, shortening and margarine increased 130%, 136%, and 410%, respectively, thanks to manufacturing. While changes in the way we work and eat reflect a society marked by prosperity and a long life expectancy, there are also less-than-fortunate ramifications.

Technology speeds on, but the biology of our bodies hasn't caught up to modern lifestyle changes. Pollution, stress, lack of physical activity, lack of adequate sleep and overconsumption of processed foods have all contributed to fairly recent health developments, such as the introduction of long-term chronic illnesses that are now the top causes of death.

Furthermore, these conditions — heart disease, cancer, lung disease, dementia — start around midlife and create an unprecedented burden for individuals, families and societies. That means more years of coping with chronic disease. Chronic disease can wreak havoc on your quality of life. It can decrease productivity, chip away at independence and diminish social engagement.

In other words, if you develop a chronic disease such as high blood pressure, chronic obstructive pulmonary disease or diabetes, not only is your life span shortened, but the quality of life you do have is diminished significantly.

WHAT I'VE LEARNED

After I developed my second cancer before age 40, I was convinced that cancer was going to be my cause of death and that it would likely occur much too early in my life. When I had my second cancer, our children were still quite young — Emily was 8, Katy 6, and Ben only 2 years old. I wanted to be able to watch them grow up. I wanted to grow old with my wife and enjoy many years together.

Being so sure that cancer was going to kill me — and equally convinced that I would have a premature death — I felt compelled to learn all that I could about how to prevent that from happening. My goal was to find out what my risk factors for cancer were and change them for the better as much as I could.

By the way, a risk factor is a trait or behavior that increases your risk of injury or disease. It's similar to the way that driving without a seat belt increases your risk of being injured if you're in a car wreck, or that standing next to a flagpole during an electrical storm increases your risk of being hit by lightning.

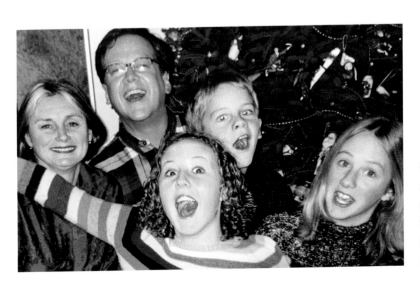

Celebrating Christmas at the end of the millennium, as well as five years of remission after I was treated for cancer the second time.

What I learned over a period of a few years was actually very surprising to me and can be summarized in two sentences. First, the risk factors for cancer are essentially the same as the risk factors for heart attack, stroke, Alzheimer's disease, diabetes, high blood pressure and erectile dysfunction. Second, I probably was not going to die of cancer but more likely of heart disease, like so many other people.

The reason I wrote this book is that it doesn't have to be this way. We can all make small changes over time to reduce our chances of chronic illness or dying prematurely.

I started this chapter off with a quote from Sir Richard Doll, a British physician and researcher who was one of the first scientists to link smoking to cancer: "Death in old age is inevitable, but death before old age is not."

YOUNG AT HEART, LITERALLY

At Mayo Clinic, we have a new software program that uses artificial intelligence to analyze electrocardiogram (ECG) results. An ECG is a common heart test that records the electrical pulses that make the heart beat. The program compares your results with large amounts of networked data and calculates your heart age versus your chronological age. The healthier your heart, the younger your ECG heart age. Obviously, you would like your heart age to be younger than your chronological age. This would mean that you've been taking care of yourself and doing all the right things to minimize the aging process.

Among cancer survivors, heart age is typically older than chronological age. One reason for this is that the risk factors for heart disease and cancer are often the same — such as smoking, obesity and older age. Also, cancer treatments such as radiation can promote coronary artery disease if the heart is in the radiation field, as mine was. Chemotherapy, which I also received, can affect the heart muscle so that it doesn't pump and relax as effectively as it should.

A report from the Centers for Disease Control and Prevention found that men who survived cancer had a heart age 8.5 years older than the heart age of men who'd never had cancer. Women cancer survivors had a heart age 6.5 years older than the heart age of women with no prior cancer. For men over 60 with a history of cancer, as I am, heart age was likely to be 15 years older than chronological age.

I want to live for as long as I can. Having cancer twice really put that goal into sharp focus for me. But it's also not enough for me to just simply live longer. I want to live longer in good health, so that I can enjoy a long life with my wife and children. I want to be able to enjoy retirement one day. I want to enjoy playing with grandchildren in the future. I want to be free to travel and do many things.

When I first started in medicine, it wasn't clear to me how to accomplish this. But during my career at Mayo Clinic, I've learned a few things. I've shared this knowledge with my patients, with my friends and family, and now, in this book, I share it with you. So let's put a spin on Doll's words, shall we? Yes, death is inevitable. But premature death or growing old with a chronic disease is not.

For these reasons, I was quite concerned about what my heart age would be at age 65, more than 20 years after my last cancer treatments. But instead of being 8.5 years older, my heart age was actually 17 years younger — a difference of more than 25 years compared with what was expected. We'll talk in the remainder of the book about what I've done and what I've learned that can help you have a younger heart.

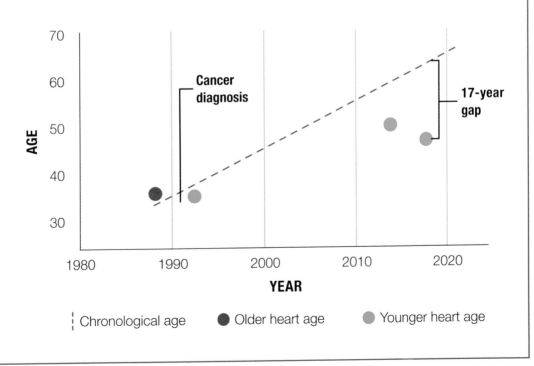

"IT IS UNFORTUNATE THAT SO FEW APPRECIATE FROM WHAT SMALL CAUSES DISEASES COME."

— cofounder of Mayo Clinic Dr. Charles H. Mayo

CHAPTER 2

How do we get from healthy to diseased?

Most of us are born in relatively good health. And unless we develop a childhood illness, we grow into our young adult lives without too many trips to the doctor. Most untimely deaths in those under age 45 are caused by things that can't be controlled, like accidents. In that sense, I was a bit of an outlier when I developed cancer as a young adult.

As we get older, though, what strips us of our health and eventually our lives are conditions that affect us over the long term, chronic diseases of the heart and blood vessels, diabetes, dementia and other illnesses that are common today.

How does it happen? How do we become ill? Or more importantly, how do we stay healthy? How do we keep our bodies from wearing down too soon and becoming increasingly susceptible to disease?

HEALTH DOESN'T EXIST IN A VACUUM

The truth is, our health doesn't exist in a vacuum. It results from a complex interplay between what's going on inside our bodies and what's happening outside of them in the environment.

Human beings have a dynamic internal system that shifts and responds to triggers from the environment. The outside world contains a host of health challenges — from microscopic viral invaders to sweeping tsunamis and hurricanes.

Every moment of every day, our bodies are working hard to keep our internal systems in balance and ready to adapt to change. But if our defenses are undermined and internal systems become unbalanced, illness and disease can occur.

How do our internal systems become unbalanced? The body's internal harmony (homeostasis) can be disrupted by a number of factors, some of them within our control, some not.

Internal malfunctions, such as genetic mutations, are often beyond our control. The wear and tear on our organs and blood vessels due to aging is also somewhat inevitable.

But today's leading causes of death aren't generated primarily by internal malfunctions. More often, they're brought on by our interactions with the world around us. Luckily, many of us have a lot of control over these exchanges.

Internal malfunctions

Every so often, diseases occur because of something going wrong with the body's genetic code — a DNA malfunction. For example, certain inherited genetic mutations are known to cause specific diseases, some of which can be fatal. Huntington's disease is a rare yet devastatingly straightforward example of an illness caused by a single genetic mutation.

Other times, genetic variations aren't a direct cause of disease, but they create vulnerabilities that predispose people to certain kinds of illnesses. For example, some people are born with a genetic predisposition to certain types of breast cancer or to an autoimmune disorder such as celiac disease that makes them allergic to gluten.

Even more-common illnesses, such as heart disease and diabetes, have been linked to genetic variants called single nucleotide polymorphisms (SNPs). Individually, these small genetic variations don't cause harm, but together they can increase a person's chances of developing a certain disease.

An example of this is something as simple as your blood type. If your blood type is A or B, your risk of heart attack is increased approximately 20% compared with someone who has blood type O. If your blood type is AB, your risk of heart attack is increased 40%. This doesn't mean that a heart attack is definitely in your future, only that your risk is increased.

Genes play a smaller part in our health than we might think. All told, genetics accounts for maybe 20% of overall health. Thinking back to my sister's experience with breast cancer and my own double bout with cancer, I reflected that even if I did have a genetic tendency toward the disease, it was not a fait accompli, so to speak. There was more to my health puzzle than just genetics.

While we cannot change our genes, we can certainly modify how our bodies express our genes by altering our lifestyles.

Everyday interactions

Most often, our health is compromised because of our interactions with the world around us. Some external factors — such as accidents, infections or even intentional self-harm — can damage our health and sometimes kill us. But factors such as these account for maybe another 20% of overall health.

Access to health care also affects our health. Some people have less access to health care services than others, perhaps because of lack of funds or resources, inadequate medical insurance, or reduced proximity to medical offices and hospitals. But access to health care services accounts for only about 10% of overall health.

So what about the other 50%? You are the biggest driver of your own health. Your daily behaviors are the single most important factor in keeping you healthy. While certain genetic variations may indeed increase a person's risk of heart attack, a lifestyle that includes things like smoking, eating unhealthy foods, sitting too much and not exercising can increase that person's risk of a heart attack by 400%!

In today's modern society, the way in which we interact with our environment — our behaviors combined with circumstances — have an oversized effect on our health compared with genetics.

It's true that for plenty of us, our circumstances may not always be ideal or under our control. But at the same time, it's heartening to know that making healthy choices in our daily lives can play a huge role in keeping our internal systems in balance and healthy.

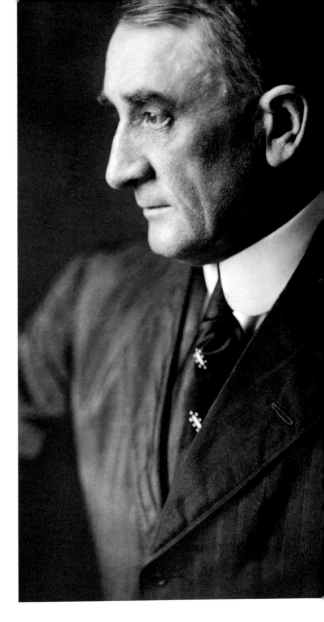

Dr. Charles H. Mayo (above), one of the co-founders of Mayo Clinic, said, "It is unfortunate that so few appreciate from what small causes diseases come." This idea is so true today. Diseases really do come from all of the tiny, seemingly inconsequential decisions we make every day. But eventually, these decisions take their toll.

Death by a thousand cuts

It's tempting to think that personal health tends to decline all at once. To be honest, that's how most of us probably perceive illness. We're not aware of the small, silent changes going on inside of our bodies until a heart attack happens or a tumor becomes noticeable. When the diagnosis hits, it feels like it's the diagnosis that has put us over the health precipice and sent us careening onto a path we didn't anticipate.

"I'd be fine If I just wouldn't have had that single episode of illness." I hear this often from my patients. That single episode might be an infection, a heart attack, a blood clot in the lungs or something else that led to a series of other medical problems.

Although we often see illness as a single event, it's no more of a single event than is wealth. You may see a businesswoman who has a nice car, house or other signs of wealth. But unless she won the lottery, which is extremely rare, she probably acquired these things through many years of steady work.

In the same way, disease often develops over many years. For example, a heart attack, in most cases, is the culmination of years of chronic inflammation in the arteries (see "Artery inflammation" on the next page). The blood vessel lining (endothelium) gradually develops a small area of damage, which leads to a blood clot. The clot can close off the artery like a cork in a bottle, cutting off blood supply to the heart and causing a heart attack. Amazingly, almost

half of all heart attacks occur because of a blood clot lodging in an artery that's only mildly narrowed.

Likewise, we're typically not aware of cancer cells growing in our bodies until a test reveals them or a tumor forms and signs and symptoms appear. Often, the growth of a tumor takes years to develop. Even Alzheimer's disease is now known to develop over many years, even decades, before symptoms appear.

Most chronic diseases develop over time as the result of a buildup of small detrimental changes inside the body. One small plaque in a blood vessel likely won't kill you. But a long-term buildup of plaques can. The good news is that this slow pathway presents an opportunity to stop and even reverse the progression of disease.

A LOOK INSIDE

What are these small detrimental changes in the body that lead to chronic illness? Although scientists are still exploring the mechanisms for many chronic illnesses, a common thread that appears to run through almost all of them — and a source of intrigue and fascination to many scientists — is a subtle state of low-grade chronic inflammation.

Chronic irritation

Inflammation is part of the body's natural defense process designed to protect against things like infections, toxins and trauma, and to repair any damage that might occur. The inflammatory response activates a cascade of immune reactions that eliminates germs and repairs injured cells. For example, if you nick your finger, you'll notice fairly quickly that the area around the wound becomes red and inflamed. This is a sign that the immune system has been activated and is sending immune cells to clean up the area and knit the skin back together.

But scientists have also noticed that a low-grade form of inflammation can occur on a whole-body (systemic) level. This type of inflammation can occur in response to things

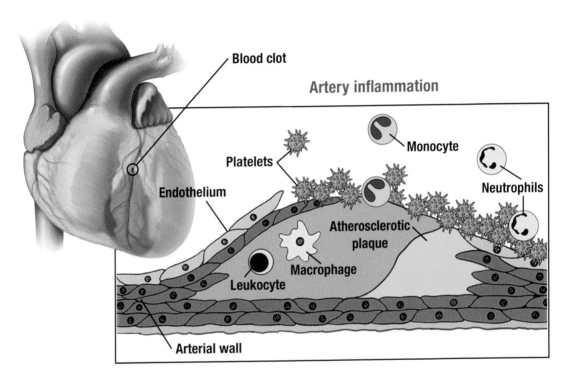

The **endothelium**, a thin layer of cells lining the inside of your arteries, can be damaged by multiple causes, including things like smoking, high blood pressure and a poor diet. The damage activates the body's immune system, bringing in immune cells (**leukocytes, macrophages, monocytes** and **neutrophils**) in an attempt to repair the **arterial wall**. Blood cells (**platelets**) also clump at the injury site. The resulting inflammation, often chronic, creates an environment that promotes the buildup of **atherosclerotic plaques**, which narrow the artery and restrict blood flow. Sometimes a **blood clot** forms, blocking blood flow to the heart and causing a heart attack.

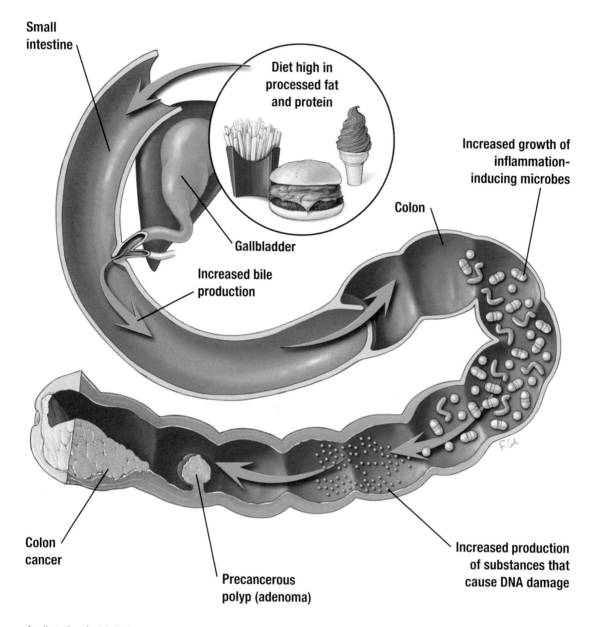

Small intestine

Diet high in processed fat and protein

Gallbladder

Increased bile production

Colon

Increased growth of inflammation-inducing microbes

Increased production of substances that cause DNA damage

Colon cancer

Precancerous polyp (adenoma)

A diet that's high in **processed fat and protein** can increase your risk of colon cancer through a gradual series of events. To digest fat and protein molecules, your **gallbladder** produces additional bile. **Increased bile** in the colon alters the balance of **microbes** in the **colon,** causing continuous low-level inflammation and production of substances than can harm the genetic sequences (DNA) of your intestinal cells. This **DNA damage** can lead to a disorganized growth of cells **(adenoma),** which can eventually develop into **colon cancer**.

like a steady diet of saturated fats and little fiber or to continuously high stress levels. This constant state of low-grade inflammation loses its initial purpose of inducing healing and leads instead to increased cellular and tissue damage. It becomes a source of chronic irritation to tissues in the body, and eventually it becomes a problem. One example is acid reflux. We all have very strong acid in our stomachs, which is

CAN A DISEASE BE REVERSED?

Although our bodies are capable of generating new cells for certain tasks, such as new immune cells or fresh blood cells, the bodies we are born with are the ones we have for life. Once tissues have been damaged by injury or disease, it's tough to reverse that damage (or else we'd be like self-healing superheroes). But it is possible to reverse some disease progression.

An example is coronary artery disease. Coronary artery disease develops when the major blood vessels that supply your heart become damaged and diseased. Cholesterol-containing deposits (atherosclerotic plaques) in your coronary arteries along with inflammation are usually to blame for coronary artery disease.

The coronary arteries supply blood, oxygen and nutrients to your heart. A buildup of plaques can damage and narrow these arteries, decreasing blood flow to your heart. Eventually, the reduced blood flow may cause chest pain (angina), shortness of breath, or other coronary artery disease signs and symptoms. A complete blockage can cause a heart attack.

It's not possible to make the damaged arteries like new again, but it is possible to make it easier for blood to flow through them. Soft plaques that have accumulated in the arteries can be cleared away by eating more anti-inflammatory foods (such as fruits, vegetables and olive oil), using cholesterol-lowering drugs, and taking steps to limit additional artery damage from smoking, chronic stress and high blood pressure.

So although we can't completely reverse damage done by disease, we can reverse some of its processes and limit additional damage.

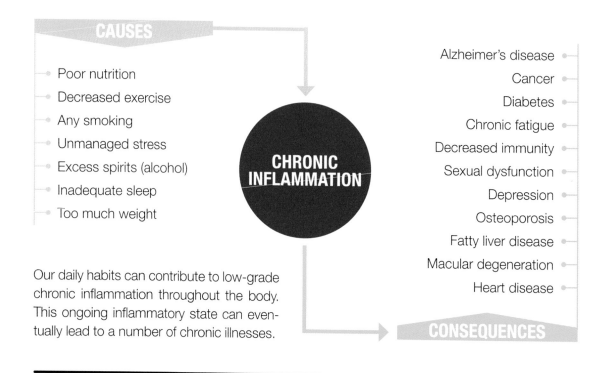

CAUSES

- Poor nutrition
- Decreased exercise
- Any smoking
- Unmanaged stress
- Excess spirits (alcohol)
- Inadequate sleep
- Too much weight

Alzheimer's disease
Cancer
Diabetes
Chronic fatigue
Decreased immunity
Sexual dysfunction
Depression
Osteoporosis
Fatty liver disease
Macular degeneration
Heart disease

CHRONIC INFLAMMATION

Our daily habits can contribute to low-grade chronic inflammation throughout the body. This ongoing inflammatory state can eventually lead to a number of chronic illnesses.

CONSEQUENCES

necessary to start the breakdown of foods we eat and to ensure that no bacteria get through to our small intestines. Sometimes, this acid can flow back (reflux) into the lower end of the gullet (esophagus). Acid doesn't bother the stomach much since it produces it and is used to it. However, the esophagus doesn't have the protective barrier that the stomach has. Acid in the esophagus can cause the pain that many know as acid reflux or gastroesophageal reflux disease (GERD).

Acid reflux is a form of inflammation. This inflammatory response is typically temporary and resolves once the acid is no longer flowing backward and the esophageal tissue is healing. But repeated bouts of acid reflux over time, as in the case of GERD, can lead to more-serious problems such as cancer of the tissues in the esophagus.

Why is inflammation so bad?

Isn't inflammation just a normal response to an injury — isn't it part of the body's self-repair system when damage occurs? Yes, inflammation is a way that the body can repair itself. But inflammation is supposed to be a temporary response. If it's ongoing, it can be damaging.

Consider tuberculosis, an infectious disease that occurs in the lungs. The immune system responds to the inflammation caused by this infection by building a wall (Ghon complex) around the infectious organism. The Ghon complex grows quite large, crowding and pressing against normal lung tissue. This wall impairs healthy tissue function and increases the risk of further infection.

Or sometimes the inflammation response involves the need for the body to repair its tissues and grow new cells. New cell growth requires massive amounts of DNA replication. If just one step in the replication process goes wrong and the DNA is altered (mutated), this could lead to abnormal cell growth or cancer. Eating too much red meat, for example, or even smaller amounts of processed meat, can cause a state of chronic inflammation, which can lead to DNA mutations that can then lead to colon cancer.

One of the most damaging examples of chronic inflammation, however, is a mild elevation of blood pressure. Blood pressure is measured in millimeters of mercury (mmHg) and appears as one number over another, like this: 120/80 mmHg. (Mercury is a substance heavier than blood. The greater the millimeters in the measurement, the higher the blood pressure.)

The top number of the blood pressure measurement indicates the systolic phase of the heartbeat. This is when the heart contracts and pumps blood out. Blood flowing out provides oxygen and nourishment to all of the body's tissues and carries waste products back for elimination from the body.

The bottom number of the blood pressure measurement reflects the diastolic phase, when the heart supposedly rests. I say supposedly because that's what most people assume, and diastole is often called the relaxation phase. However, the heart never really rests. It's more like a rubber band. It requires energy to pull a rubber band back, but once you let go it quickly contracts to resume its original form, which is its lowest energy state.

The heart beats about 100,000 times a day. At this rate, even mild increases in blood pressure can cause problems over time. Current guidelines consider a normal blood pressure to be at or below 120/80 mmHg. But, in most cases, treatment is only recommended once blood pressure is greater than 130/80 mmHg because there are side effects to treatment.

My patients frequently ask: Do I have to treat my blood pressure? It's only a little high (for example, 134/82 mmHg). But if you multiply even mild elevations of blood pressure by 100,000 times a day — which means the heart beats 1 billion times over a period of about 27 years — your risk of stroke and heart attack is significantly increased over time.

Why? Higher blood pressure damages the lining of the arteries (endothelium). The endothelium is like wallpaper but much more dynamic. It's a single-cell layer that's metabolically active — it tells the muscle deeper in the artery when to contract and relax. Contracting the muscle increases the blood pressure and relaxing the muscle decreases it.

Damage to the endothelium from high blood pressure kicks off inflammation in an attempt at repair. Eventually, this inflammatory cycle of damage and repair leads to a thickened endothelium and narrowed artery.

High blood pressure also accelerates the buildup of fatty deposits in your arteries (atherosclerosis). When the endothelium is damaged, blood cells and fat cells often clump together at the injury site. They invade and scar deeper layers of the artery walls. Large accumulations of these fatty deposits are called plaques.

Over time the plaques harden and further narrow the arteries. Organs and tissues served by these narrowed arteries don't get an adequate supply of blood. Your heart responds by increasing the pressure to maintain adequate blood flow. The increased pressure leads to further blood vessel damage, which leads to more inflammation.

The higher pressure of blood running through the arteries 100,000 times a day leads to this damage of the endothelium. Chronic inflammation of the endothelium is a leading global problem because it contributes to heart attacks and strokes.

Causes of chronic inflammation

Increasing evidence suggests that chronic inflammation is tied to multiple factors surrounding our daily habits. These factors include:

Physical inactivity When skeletal muscles contract during physical activity, they release proteins into the bloodstream that help to reduce inflammation throughout the body. Inactive muscles, on the other hand, lead to an increase in pro-inflammatory molecules — a trend seen not only in breast cancer survivors and people with diabetes but also in healthy people. Numerous studies have shown an inverse relationship between physical activity and measures of inflammation — in other words, the greater the amount of physical activity, the lower the level of inflammation. Even short bouts of exercise are known to have anti-inflammatory effects.

Unhealthy diet Eating an unbalanced diet can lead to chronic inflammation. A diet that's low in fruits, vegetables and whole grains and high in sodium, alcohol, trans fats and ultraprocessed foods can change the composition of your gut microbiome, among other things. The gut microbiome is made up of all of the microorganisms — including bacteria, fungi, viruses and other tiny organisms — that normally live in your digestive tract and contribute to internal homeostasis. An upset in the balance of these microorganisms can ultimately lead to low-grade inflammation.

Obesity Both diet and activity levels contribute to obesity, which is also linked to changes in the gut microbiome and inflammation. Excessive abdominal fat (visceral adipose tissue) is an important trigger of inflammation. The tissue itself is an active organ with molecular processes of its own.

These processes kick off certain chemical chain reactions that result in a proliferation of pro-inflammatory molecules and substances. Over time, inflammation can become chronic and cause damage.

Stress and sleep disturbance Persistent stress tends to disrupt the sensitive link between hormone production and the immune system's ability to regulate inflammation. Extended periods of stress can lead to a chronic uptick in inflammation. Prolonged lack of quality sleep also can lead to a sustained activation of inflammatory pathways and contribute to chronic systemic inflammation.

Environmental and industrial pollutants With the rapid expansion of cities and industrial areas in modern society, our exposure to air pollutants, hazardous waste products and industrial chemicals has increased exponentially. Thousands of chemicals exist in the world today but only a small portion have been evaluated for their health effects.

Of those chemical that have been evaluated, a number of them are commonly used and have been linked to inflammatory processes in the body. In addition, there is clear evidence that pollutants such as tobacco smoke can damage our lungs and airways, leading to lung cancer and chronic lung disease. Direct inhalation of tobacco smoke can cause serious damage, but lingering harmful effects have been shown for second- and third-hand smoke, as well (see Chapter 12).

WHICH WAY FORWARD?

At the end of the day, it isn't always clear why one person gets cancer or another has a heart attack or stroke or develops Alzheimer's disease. But it does appear that similar inflammatory processes contribute to these seemingly very different diseases.

The good news is that we can modify many of the factors that contribute to chronic inflammation — such as sleep, stress, physical activity and diet — to minimize its effects on our bodies. By doing so, we also reduce our risk of developing serious chronic illnesses, and we increase the length of time we live in good health without these diseases. In other words, we increase our "health span," which is the topic of the next chapter.

MOST OF US SPEND A DECADE OF OUR LIVES WITH A CHRONIC ILLNESS THAT'S IN MANY WAYS PREVENTABLE.

CHAPTER 3

A longer life in good health

I frequently tell my patients that I would like them to live 100 years and be in the nursing home, in a wheelchair and living with dementia for only the last three days of their lives, not the last decade. I want them to have a long life span but also a long health span. My patients like that concept — often times they will tell me, "Why stop at 100, doc? Let's shoot for longer!"

While a life span counts the whole of our days, a health span counts how many of those days include good health. Health span is the length of time in which you go about your daily routine alert, engaged and active, before chronic conditions like heart disease or dementia make life more difficult.

When my father was born in 1909, the average American's life span was around 46 years. In the early 1900s, life span and health

span were about the same. If you lived 46 years, you'd have good health and the ability to get up and engage in your life for most of those years.

Fast forward 100 years. Americans born in 2000 can now reasonably expect to live around 75 years. That's a 63% increase in life span — or about a one-year increase for every three years between 1900 and 2000.

But while life span has dramatically increased, health span hasn't really kept pace. Yes, people are living longer — but their health is not keeping up with their longevity. In fact, the gap between the average life span and the average health span is now over a decade and widening.

Because of this gap, someone may reasonably live to be 90 years old, but the last 10 or

GAP BETWEEN LIFE SPAN AND HEALTH SPAN

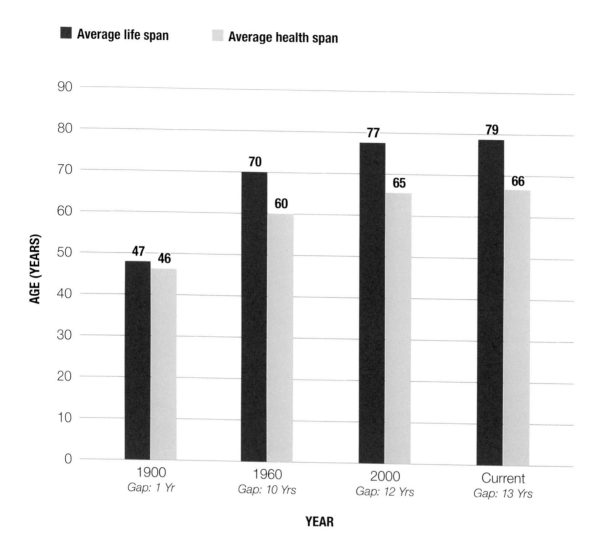

Life span is the number of years of life. Health span is the period of life spent in good health, free from the chronic diseases and disabilities of aging. Developing lifelong healthy habits is key to minimizing the gap between the two.

Based on Centers for Disease Control and Prevention, American Heart Association and other sources.

more years of life may be spent in a bed, in a nursing home or with dementia. For many, this isn't much of a life — and it's certainly not the life they'd dreamed of living.

MEASURING THE GAP

Chronic diseases and conditions are the biggest reason for a decreased health span. Heart disease, lung cancer, chronic obstructive pulmonary disease (COPD) and diabetes are the top causes of years lived with poor health.

Plenty of adults in the U.S. have chronic illnesses. According to the Rand Corp., a nonprofit research organization, approximately 60% of American adults live with at least one chronic condition, the most common of which is high blood pressure (a key risk factor for heart disease and diabetes). About 40% of U.S. adults have more than one chronic illness and over 10% has five or more chronic conditions.

Chronic illnesses tend to multiply with age. Over 80% of Americans 65 and older have multiple chronic illnesses. But even among middle-age people, around half have multiple chronic illnesses.

Not only does having a chronic illness decrease your health span, it also decreases life expectancy. A 2014 study of Medicare beneficiaries found that life expectancy decreased for *each* additional chronic illness a person had, ranging from almost six months for the first chronic illness to around 2.5 years for the sixth condition.

THE COST OF CHRONIC ILLNESS

Chronic illness imposes not only physical and mental burdens but also a financial one. The vast majority of health care spending in the U.S. is on treating chronic illnesses. According to the Centers for Disease Control and Prevention, 90% of the country's $3.5 trillion in annual health care spending is on chronic and mental health conditions.

Take diabetes, for example. Type 2 diabetes is a common chronic condition in the U.S. and accounts for the vast majority of diabetes cases. It happens when your body becomes resistant to the effects of insulin and doesn't process blood sugar the way it should. In 2017, nearly 10% of American adults had a diagnosis of diabetes.

Type 2 diabetes can be easy to ignore, especially in the early stages when you're feeling fine. Although the disease process is slow, it's insidious. Eventually, diabetes can have many complications. It can dramatically increase your risk of heart disease, stroke, high blood pressure and narrowed blood vessels. It can cause loss of feeling in your toes and fingers. It can cause kidney failure and glaucoma. It can make you more susceptible to skin infections, and it may even increase your risk of Alzheimer's disease.

Diabetes is one of the most expensive chronic illnesses in America. The average cost per year for a person with diabetes in 2017 was close to $10,000. This includes direct costs, such as insulin, medications, doctor visits,

4 COMMON END-OF-LIFE HEALTH PATTERNS

There are four common ways for human life to end. Most of us would prefer to live in full control of our physical capabilities for as long as possible before we die. The most effective way for us to achieve this outcome is to practice healthy habits throughout our lives — good nutrition, plenty of exercise, adequate rest, reduced stress, limited alcohol, no smoking and a healthy weight.

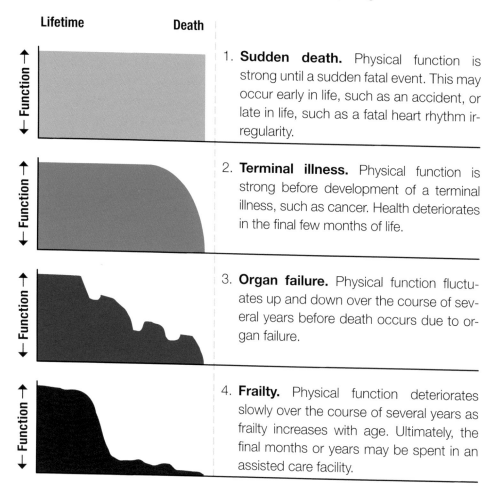

Lifetime   **Death**

1. **Sudden death.** Physical function is strong until a sudden fatal event. This may occur early in life, such as an accident, or late in life, such as a fatal heart rhythm irregularity.

2. **Terminal illness.** Physical function is strong before development of a terminal illness, such as cancer. Health deteriorates in the final few months of life.

3. **Organ failure.** Physical function fluctuates up and down over the course of several years before death occurs due to organ failure.

4. **Frailty.** Physical function deteriorates slowly over the course of several years as frailty increases with age. Ultimately, the final months or years may be spent in an assisted care facility.

Based on *JAMA*. 2003;289:2387.

home health care and hospital care. It doesn't include indirect costs such as missing work, not being able to perform as well on the job or not working at all. And it doesn't include the costs in terms of pain, dissatisfaction and decreased quality of life.

What are two of the biggest factors that put you at risk of type 2 diabetes? Weight and physical inactivity — factors closely linked to daily habits.

Lifestyle effects

Clearly, American adults aren't in very good health, especially as they get older. And people in other countries, both developed and developing ones, are following a similar storyline. How did we find ourselves in a global epidemic of chronic disease?

As we examined in the last chapter, most chronic illnesses affecting people today are actually lifestyle illnesses. In other words, these diseases are rooted in our daily activities, in the choices we make each and every day. And these daily choices contribute to widespread changes in the body, such as chronic inflammation, which eventually take their toll. What are some of these pro-inflammatory activities?

More sitting Sitting has become prevalent in American society. Many people work in front of a computer at a desk all day, then come home and relax on the couch while watching TV. They may spend 10, 11, or even 12 or more hours a day sitting.

Why is sitting bad for us? Because our bodies are programmed to move frequently (every hour or so) throughout the day. Low physical activity encourages inflammation.

This sedentary lifestyle has become a true health problem. Research has linked sitting for long periods with a number of health problems, including cardiovascular disease, obesity, high blood pressure, abnormal cholesterol levels, high blood sugar and cancer — all secondary to underlying inflammation.

Increased processed foods and calories Research shows that ultraprocessed foods account for almost 60% of the calories and 90% of the added sugars in a typical American diet. And, along with restaurant meals, processed foods account for about 70% of the sodium in an American diet. The result is an increased risk of high blood pressure, stroke, heart failure, obesity, kidney disease and more. In fact, in the most recent report on the state of health in the U.S., experts listed diet as the No. 1 risk factor for premature death among American adults, primarily related to heart disease.

Less rest Nearly 40% of adults surveyed reported being so tired that they fall asleep during the day without meaning to at least once per month. Sleep allows your body to rejuvenate itself and heal damaged cells and tissues. Persistent lack of sleep prevents these processes. Ongoing sleep deficiency can downgrade your immune system. It has been linked to an increased risk of heart disease, kidney disease, high blood pressure, obesity, diabetes and stroke.

More stress To many people, chronic stress feels like a normal or even necessary part of modern life. They think that something so common and universal can't be all that bad. After all, everyone they know is exposed to stress every day. But long-term activation of the stress response system and overexposure to cortisol and other stress hormones can disrupt key body processes. It can increase your risk of anxiety, depression, insomnia, weight gain, high blood pressure, heart disease and stroke.

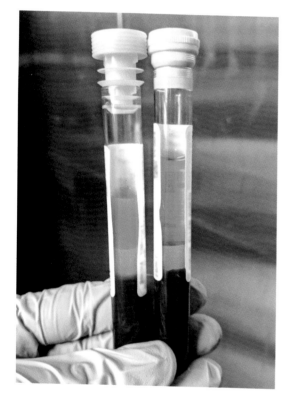

Adding a teaspoon of sugar every day to your car's fuel tank will ruin the engine. Regularly eating saturated fats will clog up your bloodstream with cholesterol (see sample on left).

Lack of support In addition, a lack of social support can lead to isolation and loneliness — which are associated with a greater risk of cardiovascular disease, high blood pressure, a weakened immune system and other health problems.

Spent money, lost time

Americans spend a lot of money and lose a lot of precious time treating chronic illness. But wouldn't it better if illness could be prevented in the first place? Wouldn't it make more sense to invest in living better now so that you can continue to live better later?

Maintaining your body is similar to maintaining a car. You need to pay attention and make good choices to avoid problems. For example, if you continually hit potholes, eventually you'll either get a flat tire or the wheels will go out of alignment on your car. Driving with low or dirty oil will likely lead to engine damage. Putting in the wrong kind of fuel such as diesel instead of gasoline will lead to motor problems. All of these choices affect your car, and it will eventually break down.

It's the same with our bodies. Too often, we dismiss the value of preventive maintenance. We frequently eat food that promotes inflammation and harms our bodies. Or we run our bodies too hard without allowing for adequate amounts of rest. In order to keep our bodies and minds running well for many years, it's important to invest in daily maintenance and upkeep.

YOUR BODY IS SIMILAR TO YOUR CAR

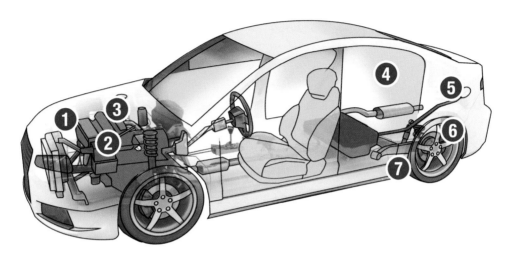

1 BATTERY = SLEEP
Recharge your battery regularly with plenty of sleep.

2 AIR FILTER = SMOKING
Keep out pollutants like tobacco that will ruin your body's engine.

3 ENGINE = EXERCISE
You use your car regularly so that the engine will work well when you need it. The same goes for regularly exercising your body.

4 WEIGHT = WEIGHT
Too much weight makes the car, and your body, work too hard and stresses its parts.

5 GAS = NUTRITION
Give your body the nutrition fuel it was designed to use. You would never put diesel fuel in an engine designed to run on gasoline.

6 BRAKES = ALCOHOL
Put the brakes on alcohol intake. Know when to stop.

7 SHOCKS/TIRES = STRESS
No road in life is without potholes. You need shock absorbers to deal with stress. You also need social support — like tires on a car — to provide balance and help you run smoothly.

TO MAKE A BIG CHANGE,
START WITH VERY SMALL STEPS.

CHAPTER 4

Slow change is permanent change

It would be really great if we all could make major lifestyle changes with a little willpower and a flip of the switch. But we might as well be honest — that expectation isn't logical or reasonable. Worse, it sets us up for disappointment and reinforces the negative mindset many of us have about our ability to change.

When we set big goals for ourselves that require sudden, drastic changes to our daily lives, those changes might last for a day or two but not much longer. We might be able to maintain an austere diet, intense fitness plan or dramatic sleep program for a while. But these extreme behaviors usually don't become enduring habits that stand the test of time. In moments of stress or exhaustion, we quickly regress to our old habits because they're easier and they're what we're used to. The next morning, we wake up with a feeling of failure that discourages us from returning to our earlier goals.

Clearly, this problem affects many people. Think of the perennial New Year's resolution. How many of us have made dramatic promises to ourselves — to get fit, lose weight, sleep better, conquer stress — only to give up by the middle of January? In fact, Jan. 17 is the average day that Americans give up on their New Year's resolutions. When we fail, most of us think, "I need more willpower," which is exactly wrong.

Think of all the people each year who join fitness centers or buy shiny new exercise equipment with the best of intentions. After years of not working out, they go full force, telling themselves that this is it — this is the year they're finally going to get into shape. What happens? After one or two workouts, they pull a muscle, strain their back or injure a joint. Hurting and discouraged, they can't bring themselves to return to the gym or step back on that fitness machine. They tell themselves, "I'm not cut out for this. Why bother?" This is one of the reasons that almost 7 out of 10 people who join a gym rarely set foot in it after the first month.

The same thing happens to many of us when we try to change our eating patterns. At any one time, nearly half of all adults in the U.S. are attempting to lose weight. By making drastic changes to their diets, many of them may succeed. But those big, sudden changes typically don't stick. Over time, most people regain the weight or gain back even more than they lost in the first place.

One thing is certain, we do need a change — a change in the way we think about the goals we set for ourselves. We need to slow down and start small — very small.

SMALL CHANGES, BIG RESULTS

In my own life and in working with my patients, I've found that the fastest way to create a lasting habit is to go slow. How can going slow be fast? Think of the moral from that old fable about the tortoise and the hare: Slow and steady wins the race. We're more likely to succeed when we make small changes over a long period of time.

Successful businesspeople intuitively understand this. They know you can't build a business in one day. Maybe you set up shop in your basement, chipping away at your goal day after day and month after month. You learn as you go, celebrate each small success and build on those successes little by little. Your transition from basement office to office building doesn't happen in one leap but with many baby steps.

Parents get it too. They know a child can't be taught everything in a day, week or year. It takes many years — and many small moments of struggle, patience and triumph — to successfully raise a child.

Successful athletes are no different. Think of a professional football team that wins the Super Bowl. If you could ask the players how long it took to prepare for that single hour of playtime, they'd tell you it took thousands of hours. Thousands of countless incremental changes to their technique, behavior and bodies added up to that big victory.

You can do this

When I give my patients recommendations to improve their health and longevity, it's generally nothing they haven't heard before: Eat healthy foods, exercise, don't smoke, get enough sleep. Unfortunately, these statements have been repeated so often that they've become impossible cliches. It seems terribly daunting to get in shape or lose weight or get a handle on smoking or stress.

Chances are, you're a lot like the people who walk through my door. You know that eating a nutritious diet and getting enough exercise are important for your health. You may know you need more sleep and less stress in your life. Perhaps you want to stop smoking and drink less alcohol too. The problem is, you don't know how to get from point A to point B. And in this, you're not alone.

Let me ask you what I ask many of my patients: What have you accomplished in your life that you're proud of? Maybe you've raised a couple of great kids or built a successful career. Maybe you've experienced success in sports or turned a hobby into a business. Maybe your big accomplishment is just surviving. No matter how you answer the question, I'm betting that you reached your goal by taking one tiny step after another over a long stretch of time. And if you've done that before, you can do it again.

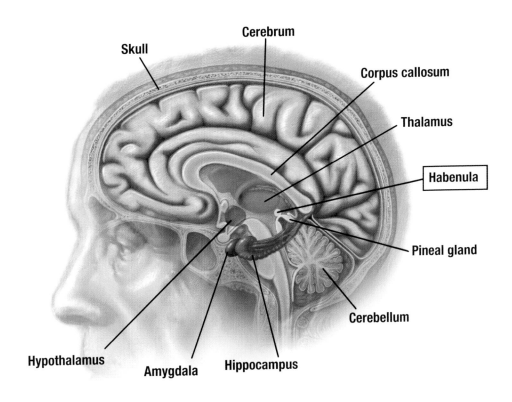

The habenula is a tiny organ located deep in the brain, near the pineal gland and the thalamus. It plays a role in guiding behavioral choices based on past experiences. Responses to unanticipated failure or lack of expected success are processed through the habenula, such that memories of a disappointing outcome trigger the impulse to adjust or avoid the behavior that led to that outcome.

What failure teaches us

When it comes to change, we often think, "Go big or go home." And if we fail, so what? Just try again. But our brains are sneaky in the way they work. And this mindset may actually work against us.

How? There's a tiny, primitive part of the brain called the habenula, which is present in most living animals. It's like the "negative reward" or "failure" center of the brain and is known for its role in shaping behavior based on past failures and disappointments (see page 45).

If you think about it, there's a reason humans evolved to have a center like this in the brain. Imagine a million years ago, a human climbed a tree to get some food but fell and broke a leg. The brain remembers the pain of that failure. It's a subconscious memory that we don't usually recognize, but it plays a big role in preventing us from experiencing repeated pain. The habenula tries to protect us from future failures by inhibiting us, sometimes even physically.

What if, on the other hand, climbing that tree resulted in finding delicious fruit to eat? That success also is ingrained in memory. Previous successes motivate us to repeat the successful action.

How does this feature of our brains impact us now? If we try to make a change but fail, the habenula records that failure. The next time we try to repeat that activity, our habenulas deter us in subtle ways. On the other hand, if we try to do something we've been successful at before, the memory of that first success enhances our chances of success the next time.

When we try to make big changes and fail, our next attempt is likely to be less successful. Unfortunately, many of us try the same change over and over only to reinforce the failure memory in the habenula. It's much better to register tiny successes than big failures in our path toward change. Once we understand this part of our brain, we can make sure the habenula works for us rather than against us.

KNOW YOUR WHY, WHAT AND HOW

Many people think that changing a behavior is all about willpower. I might say, "I'm going on a no-carb diet this month, and by gum, I'm sticking to it!" I make a strong commitment in the hope that my willpower will sustain me day after day. While such intensity may spur me on at the beginning, my willpower is unlikely to get me through more than the first few days of my new diet.

Research shows, however, that people who do have healthy habits aren't really using all that much willpower or conscious effort. On the contrary, they've learned to put their positive behaviors on autopilot, so that willpower becomes a moot point. What may begin as a conscious commitment motivated by specific goals gradually becomes behaviors they engage in without much thought or effort.

How does this shift to autopilot happen? What follows are some tips and tricks that have helped me and many of my patients establish healthy habits. By preparing and planning for a new habit — and giving ourselves time to organically grow that habit — we can set ourselves up for success.

Start with the 'why'

Successful change begins with powerful motivation, which is different from willpower. Ask yourself, "Why do I want to lose weight?" or "Why should I get more exercise?" Really think about it. Get clear about your motivation. This is the single most important factor because it helps you with the seemingly insignificant decisions you make hundreds of times a day.

In general, positive motivations are more effective than negative ones. Guilt, shame or fear won't inspire you in the long run as much as a hopeful goal will. Instead of being motivated by the fear of a heart attack, for example, you might focus your energies on the goal of seeing a grandchild graduate. Instead of focusing on a dislike of your physical appearance, you might strive to have more energy and a greater zest for life. A positive motivation — whatever it is — can be a powerful engine. A singular goal to which you're deeply committed can push you forward and keep you going as you begin to form new healthy habits.

A big part of why we fail in changing a behavior comes from not understanding and identifying our "why." When we have difficulty eating differently, being more active, or reducing unhealthy habits such as smoking or drinking too much alcohol, it's essential that we understand why we are trying to accomplish such a goal.

Take, for example, changing our eating patterns. The average American makes a couple of hundred decisions a day on eating. The decisions are usually about what to eat and how much. As the day goes on we suffer decision fatigue, which leads to decisions that we regret later.

But if you understand your "why" for changing your eating habits, it provides strong positive motivation during difficult decision times. The "why" is essential and it allows us to do the "what," the "how" and the "when."

Move on to the 'what'

Once you know why you want to make healthy changes in your life, the next step is to decide what you're going to do to make this happen. Get specific. Think about the areas in which you want or need to improve.

Focus on your habits. Our habits control at least half of what we do every day — over 50% of the calories we eat are out of habit, for example. We're often unaware of our habits and don't even remember doing them. Have you ever driven to work and not remembered the ride? You think later, "Oh my gosh, did I drive safely?"

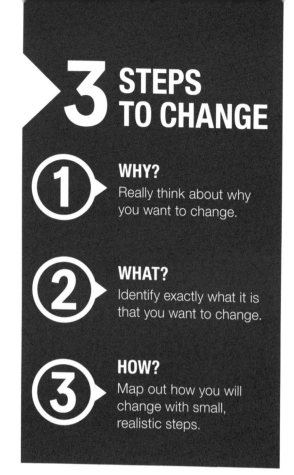

3 STEPS TO CHANGE

① WHY?
Really think about why you want to change.

② WHAT?
Identify exactly what it is that you want to change.

③ HOW?
Map out how you will change with small, realistic steps.

We do routine things without too much thought because our brains want to conserve energy, and a habit is the easiest way to do it. So changing a habit is the best way to change your lifestyle.

It's extremely helpful to know what a habit is in the first place. Knowing what a habit is, how it forms and then controls our actions, makes it more likely that we can modify habits for the better. The term *habit* has been defined by many people, but the best definition, I think, is by Wendy Wood from the University of Southern California. She de-

fines a habit as an action that we take, in a certain context, to gain a reward.

Here's an example. I usually get up about 5 a.m., quietly, so as to not awaken my wife, Linda. I walk into the kitchen (context), and without even thinking, I make a cup of coffee (action) to get a warm delicious coffee with a wonderful aroma (reward). The reward is key, and it needs to be immediate. When I get the reward, my brain releases dopamine, which helps lay down the memory for this habit. The reason the reward needs to be immediate is so that the memory links the context and the action with the reward.

Figure out the 'how'

The "how" of changing habits is where many of us get stuck. We tend to set vast, lofty goals for ourselves that sound good on paper: We'll lose 50 pounds, train for a marathon or master meditation. The problem with these big goals is that they're often unrealistic. We end up failing and feeling defeated, something our habenulas are bound to remember. Instead, it's important to break our "how" into manageable microsteps.

Set small goals Imagine for a moment that you're teaching math to a 5-year-old child. You wouldn't tell this young student to sit down and tackle trigonometry. You'd start with basic math skills — recognizing numbers and counting them in order. You'd build on that knowledge one step at a time over many weeks, months and years.

Or say you wanted to learn to play a musical instrument, maybe the piano. Would you start with a beautiful but complex Beethoven sonata, or would you try to learn the chords first? Of course, you would try the latter.

The same process applies when you're planning to change your behavior and create new habits. You'll be more successful if you start with small steps that match both your motivation and your ability. If you've been leading a sedentary lifestyle and want to improve your fitness levels, it won't work very well to set a goal of running a mile every morning. A more realistic and likely successful goal might be to forgo the elevator at work and take the stairs each morning to your fourth-floor office. Even taking the elevator to the third floor and walking the last flight of stairs is a good beginning.

Keep in mind that no goal is too small. For example, one study found that replacing just half a tablespoon of margarine, mayonnaise or butter a day in your diet with the same amount of olive oil can help reduce your risk of heart disease.

When you set goals that you can easily attain, your confidence will grow and you'll be able to build on your success incrementally. Keep it simple. Lower the bar so that you can get some early successes and build on them.

For many years, I had been trying to get one of my patients to start exercising on his treadmill but he could never bring himself to make it a habit. Finally, at one office visit, I suggested that he start with a very small goal: Simply stand on the treadmill for 5 minutes each day. He agreed. Six weeks later at a follow-up visit, I asked him how it went with the treadmill. To my surprise, he revealed that he had begun walking on the treadmill 30 minutes a day. He figured that since he was standing there already, he might as well start walking. That one small initial step blossomed into a healthy habit after years of resistance.

Be specific A good goal is not only realistic but specific. The smaller and more detailed, the better. If you want to improve your diet, you might start by adding a single slice of apple to your breakfast each morning. Or if you don't eat breakfast, then start with just a single slice of apple. Link these tiny changes to something you already do.

For instance, if you aim to become more physically active, you could set a goal of doing at least one pushup or situp during commercial breaks of your favorite show. To lower your stress levels, you might take three deep breaths before you open your email account. In choosing specific micro-goals you're declaring what you will do and when and how you'll do it.

Make it fun As much as possible, try to choose a new habit you want to add to your life, rather than something you feel you should do. Start with the ones that you think will give you some joy or pleasure, even if the good feeling mainly comes from a sense of accomplishment. This reward can help stimulate the dopamine release that helps form the habit memory. The more

RELY ON YOUR STRENGTHS

Many of us can be successful in one area of life but not so successful in another. One of my patients who is also a good friend, Andy Fickman, is a very confident and successful movie director whose works include "She's the Man," "Race to Witch Mountain" and many other popular films. He's agreed to share his story here.

Andy and I have talked about the difficulties of shooting a movie and all the daily setbacks that occur. We discussed how he handles all the different challenges he deals with every day — personalities, schedules, budgets, weather, rewrites and much more. He told me he's developed a routine approach that no matter what happens today, he adapts and gets it done tomorrow. I asked him if he learned this approach on the first day he was shooting his first movie. His reply was, "Oh gosh, no, Doctor – it took me years to learn this!"

However, when he tried to change to a healthier diet and incorporate regular physical activity into his day, he wasn't successful. He'd often get discouraged and just try the same approach the next day, only to fail again. He didn't realize he was leaving the problem-solving skills he'd acquired in moviemaking completely untapped.

Once he realized that he could take what he learned from directing movies and apply it to things like diet and exercise, his world changed. He started applying his approach of adapting and overcoming to the challenges of healthy eating and exercising while on set. He gradually built his small daily successes into a long-term goal accomplishment.

Reflecting on what worked for him, he told me, "I have certainly tried diets and fads over the years, but none connected with me." He said that he had a little success with one particular program but found that it had everything to do with the fantastic woman running the program. When he moved and tried the same program at another location, his interest faded and he had a hard time with the system.

"Now that I'm doing it my way, I am trying to learn something new each day health-wise," he says. "Being responsible for my own shopping while away from home is helping to educate me — and helping me find items I really enjoy. I ask my wife a lot of questions every day about different foods and beverages, and she talks me through them. In the 40 days since I started making changes, I haven't had a day I felt hungry or deprived." In fact, it's the opposite, he says. He felt very motivated.

In addition, he established accountability by sharing his weekly weight loss with those close to him. It was a good mental step for him and a way to celebrate his success.

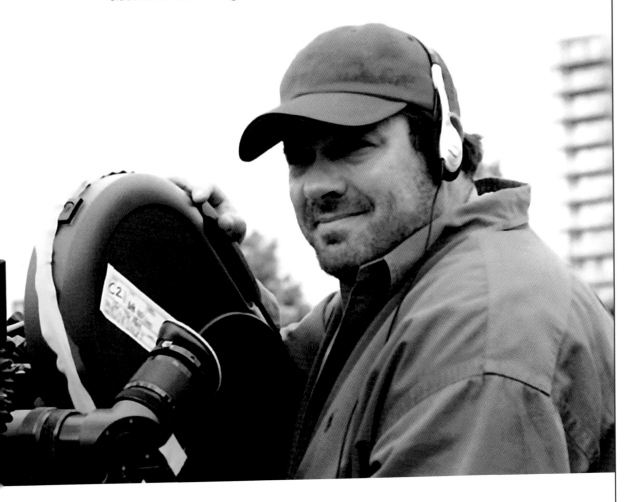

Andy Fickman on set.

you actually enjoy what you're doing, the more likely you'll stick with it.

Go slow and let it flow Once you feel confident that you're able to stick with a small, new habit, allow yourself to take the next step. It's likely you'll do this naturally, without prompting. For example, if you enjoy your morning fruit, you'll probably find it easier to cut out one bite of your breakfast bacon or egg yolks. You might find yourself doing that second and third pushup just because you can. You might extend your deep-breathing practice before reading emails to doing it before meetings or during your commute because it feels good.

TROUBLESHOOTING

What happens if you hit a wall while trying to change? We all stall out sometimes. Here are some tips to help keep you going:

- **Remember the big picture.** Keep your "why" — your central motivation — in mind when you're struggling with a new habit. Remind yourself that you're striving to live longer or set a good example for your kids. That extra serving of broccoli or weekly Zumba class represents one more step toward reaching your ultimate goal.
- **Seek support.** Changing your habits can be hard to do on your own. Many people benefit from enlisting the support of others. Vital support may come from the people closest to you, such as a spouse who agrees to help you cook healthier dinners or a friend who joins you on a weekly jog. Support might come from a community, such as a biking club for beginners. Or it could come from professionals, such as a fitness instructor or trainer, a registered dietitian, or a therapist who specializes in stress management.
- **Make it a competition.** Some people get a boost from activating their competitive streak. Joining a fitness or weight-loss challenge with a friend might be just what you need to jump-start a new habit or push you forward if you're losing steam. Just make sure that whatever challenge or competition you choose is safe, reasonable and a good match for your current level of ability.
- **Distract yourself.** New habits can be more enjoyable when you combine them with something entertaining. Stream a movie or TV show while you're sweating on the treadmill. Listen to some upbeat music when you go for a walk or run. Play an engaging podcast while you're chopping vegetables for dinner.

Be flexible If one goal isn't working, be willing to swap for a goal that does. Say, for example, you've decided to go to your local rec center every day to exercise. But you don't relish the prospect of getting dressed and driving somewhere just so you can get sweaty in public. Then change it to a different, smaller goal and link it to something you already do that you enjoy. Say you opt to exercise at home in your pajamas while watching your favorite morning show.

My wife, who is a nurse, and I often sit in the kitchen when we get home and talk about our day, which we really enjoy doing. Frequently, we'll have some cheese and maybe a beverage together. But one day we realized we were eating about 500 calories of cheese! So we decided to buy a good cheese knife so we could slice it very thin and also cut slices of apple and pear to put the cheese on. This way, we took a habit we enjoyed and made it better by eating healthy but still got the flavor of the cheese without eating as much.

TURNING ON AUTOPILOT

You already engage in countless habits every day, such as checking your email each morning, hanging up your coat after work and brushing your teeth before bed. We do these things without much thought or effort. But these automatic behaviors didn't form out of thin air. By nature, all habits are linked to some sort of cue — a time of day, setting or situation that unconsciously triggers the behavior.

A ping from your phone prompts you to pick it up and look at it. Getting out of bed in the morning cues you to turn on the shower. A dark movie theater triggers your desire for popcorn. Cues like these are powerful forces that affect how we behave throughout the day.

Knowing this can help you choose a simple cue to send a new behavior into autopilot mode. Let's say your goal is to unplug from all electronics an hour before bedtime to improve your quality of sleep. Your cue might be a specific time of night. When you see the clock strike 10, that's your cue to power down. Or maybe your goal is to graze on vegetables for your pre-dinner snack. You might decide to put a bowlful of baby carrots front and center on a shelf to greet you when you open your refrigerator.

Before embarking on a new goal, take some time to devise a cue you can easily link it to. It helps if the cue you choose is already a part of your routine. Getting out of bed, entering or leaving a room, brushing your teeth, or finishing the dishes are some examples of cues for new habits. But the possibilities are endless.

In the beginning, it will take conscious thought and effort to perform a new behavior right after a cue. You'll have to mentally remind yourself to take the stairs instead of the elevator when you first arrive at work. But with each repetition of cue plus behavior, you'll be one step closer to turning that conscious action into an automatic habit you can build on over time.

CELEBRATING SUCCESS

As you strive to establish healthy new habits, give yourself ample credit for each and every achievement. You did your five push-ups for the day? Tell yourself, "Heck, yeah!" You smoked one less cigarette? That deserves a fist pump.

By promoting the good feelings that come with practicing good habits, you'll make those habits more rewarding. And the more rewarding your brain perceives an action to be, the more you'll want to do it again (remember your habenula?).

When you make healthy choices, you start seeing yourself in a more positive light. And that has a snowball effect. The refreshed feeling that comes from getting a good night's rest might sustain your commitment to eating well throughout the day. And the sense of accomplishment you get from caring for your body in those ways could spur you to start cutting back on your smoking habit. In other words, success in one area can lead to success in another.

By the same token, a single failure doesn't mean the end of all successes. None of us is perfect. We all slip up from time to time. We skip a scheduled trip to the gym or stay up well past our bedtime. Everyone who successfully makes changes in his or her life has experienced setbacks.

It's important to keep in mind that forming new habits isn't an all-or-nothing affair. When you get off track, it doesn't mean all is lost. Remind yourself that something is better than nothing, even if it's a fraction of what you accomplished yesterday. You're still going in the right direction.

PHASING OUT OLD HABITS

So far, I've focused on how to slowly and joyfully start new habits. But what about all the old habits we want to stop? Whether we want to quit smoking, cut back on mindless snacking or stress less, old habits can be hard to change. They can feel like ingrained behaviors, an integral part of who we are and how we live.

The phrase "Break a bad habit" can be misleading. The memory of a habit lasts a lifetime. Changing an old habit takes time and must be accomplished in small steps. As Mark Twain's famous fictional character Pudd'nhead Wilson notes in his calendar, "Habit is habit and not to be flung out of the window by any man, but coaxed downstairs a step at a time."

Alter an existing habit

For example, a common habit I see is drinking a little too much alcohol, usually in social situations. Rather than tell my patients to give up alcohol altogether, I oftentimes suggest that after having the first drink, they fill the same glass with something non-alcoholic, like sparkling water. If they typically have three or four drinks at a time, I ask them to repeat the sparkling water every other drink. This cuts their alcohol intake in half with minimal effort since they're just adding to something they're already doing.

Identify cues

If you have trouble transforming old habits, don't assume that it's because you're weak or lack willpower. What's more likely is that those habits are tied to very strong cues. One of the best ways to begin phasing out an unwanted habit is to act like a detective. Start searching for the cue connected to the behavior. Notice the setting that triggers the habit you want to change.

Avoid temptation

Once you identify the cue that triggers a specific behavior, one strategy is to avoid that cue. If you grab a fistful of candy whenever you see the candy jar on your desk, get rid of the jar. If the group of smokers near the entrance to your workplace activates an urge to smoke, use an alternate entrance. If socializing at a bar leads you to drink more than you'd like, ask your friends if they can meet you at a park or coffee shop instead.

For me, I have difficulty in the morning because I love to eat crispy toast with jam on it. But this is mostly processed food that I regret eating later. The answer? I put the bread in a dark cupboard and make sure there's a bowl full of luscious-looking fruit on the kitchen counter that's easy to grab.

Change your environment

Another strategy, talked about frequently by BJ Fogg from Stanford University, is to redesign the world around you to encourage better habits. Recently, my wife and I bought this nice new refrigerator, very modern and convenient with plenty of storage and good lighting. The only problem was that the drawers for fruits and vegetables were entirely opaque. All of the healthy food we bought remained hidden and frequently forgotten. After figuring this out, we decided to put our eggs, bacon, cheese, sausage and similar foods in the opaque drawers and put the fruit and vegetables on the shelves at eye level. It really did help encourage better eating habits for us.

For persistently strong habits, try combining habit replacement with a change in your environment. If you want to stop smoking on your drive to work, replace the cigarettes with a pack of flavorful chewing gum and drive a different route to work.

Pace yourself

So choose your habits carefully. Break down the process into small, manageable steps. Alter an existing habit, gradually remove temptation and make small adjustments to your environment. Be patient with yourself as you tweak your routines little by little. Once you start to look at habits in these ways, you'll see the wisdom in the saying, "First we make our habits, then our habits make us."

GOOD HEALTH EASES STRESS, SAVES MONEY AND HELPS THE PLANET.

CHAPTER 5

Messages for millennials

Talk of chronic disease and premature death may make sense to older folks and even to some of those in their 40s and 50s. But here's the reality: Not many people in their 20s and 30s are interested nor do they feel any sense of urgency around the topic of mortality. Generally, they don't feel the need to get involved just yet.

And they're not motivated to change by statements like: "Doctors say you should do this." "You might get a heart attack one day." "You're taking years off your life."

Those are some of the most often quoted reasons to make lifestyle changes. Big, scary reasons. For many millennials, those reasons might work as a temporary jolt of fear to get a gym membership or go to bed an hour earlier. But they don't often work for long-term change.

Most millennials, generally defined as those born between 1981 and 1996, already know what they should be doing for their health in a basic sense.

"Eat healthy and get plenty of exercise" is one of the most trite, overworked expressions in use today. It's something millennials have probably been told more than once by their parents, doctors and teachers. They know to eat a healthy diet, get regular exercise, not drink too much and avoid tobacco.

Most millennials are good at practicing some healthy habits but don't do so well with others. As a generation, research shows that millennials tend to exercise more than previous generations, but they don't manage stress as well. They tend to value fruits and veggies more, but they also spend more money on processed foods.

Millennials are also facing financial challenges that affect their habits and their health. Between student debt and the rising cost of health care, many millennials are short on money and free time that could go toward gym memberships and healthy meal prep. Making healthy choices is just one of many decisions millennials face, and some have fewer resources than others. The challenges of living healthfully in a world that's not set up for it are real.

But there are good reasons — and strategies — to make changes. As a millennial, you may already face health problems of your own or of loved ones. You might be raising kids and juggling jobs while trying to make time for your own health and the health of your family. Or you might not have had time to think about your health too much yet.

Whatever your circumstances, research shows that long-term healthy habits aren't likely to result from fear, guilt or shame. The motivation to do things that are good for your body and brain — and to make those good things into habits — comes from a positive personal place. Figuring out what motivates you to make healthy changes before you hit middle age can have huge mental and physical benefits, in the long term and in the here and now.

And prioritizing health doesn't mean you need to overhaul your whole life or eat like an Instagram model every day. Healthy habits that stick are ones that fit into your life and bring benefits that you can feel, and, most importantly, are ones that you enjoy.

In this chapter we'll cover some facts about millennial health and why making changes now is a good idea. I'll also give you motivators that might actually work. Ones that are based less on guilt and more on the positive outcomes that healthy changes can bring to your life — like better mental health, more money saved and a smaller carbon footprint, to name a few. Oh, and why am I singling out millennials here? Because they're currently the largest adult generation in the U. S.

MILLENNIAL HEALTH

First — how does the health of millennials compare to the health of other generations?

You might think that people's health just keeps getting better with more medical advances and global innovation and connection. But the reality is more complicated. Because health outcomes depend so much on people's habits and environments, medical advances can't do it all. Some aspects of millennial health are getting better, while others are on the decline. And it's all subject to change.

Increase in some obesity-related cancers
Many of the cancers that are most closely linked to obesity are increasing in younger populations. Between 1995 and 2014, the rates of multiple myeloma, colorectal cancer and other obesity-related cancers went up disproportionately among young people. This rise in cancer rates can't be completely explained by increased screening.

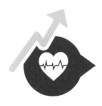

MILLENNIALS GET MORE EXERCISE

According to the Centers for Disease Control and Prevention, the percentage of people between 18 and 44 who get the recommended amount of aerobic and strength training exercise has been rising for the last 20 years. That means millennials are exercising more than previous generations did when they were younger. The millennials who get enough exercise still only make up around 30% though.

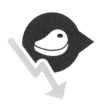

MILLENNIALS EAT LESS MEAT

They put less of their food money toward both red and white meat than any previous generation. Although the data show that as millennials' incomes go up, so does their red meat consumption. Cutting down on red meat and processed meats has been shown to have health benefits.

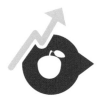

MILLENNIALS WANT TO BUY MORE FRUITS AND VEGGIES

As a whole, a bigger percentage of millennial food budgets go toward fruits and veggies than do those of Gen Xers or baby boomers. But the numbers change based on income. Millennials with lower incomes tend to spend less on produce. As incomes go up for millennials, they start to buy more fruits and veggies than previous generations. This indicates that as millennials age and their incomes go up, they'll be eating more healthy fruits and veggies than previous generations.

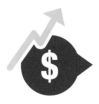

MILLENNIALS SPEND MORE ON SUGARY AND PROCESSED FOODS

The numbers show that millennials tend to buy more convenience foods. They eat out more and cook less. They also buy more sugary treats and processed foods that take little time to prepare.

Decrease in other cancers The rates of Kaposi sarcoma, cancers of the esophagus, larynx, lungs, bladder and cervix, and some other cancers are decreasing in younger people. That's especially true for cancers related to tobacco use.

Increase in risk factors for heart disease High blood pressure and diabetes, two important risk factors for heart disease, are rising disproportionately among younger people. And as of 2016, 1 in 4 young adults had prediabetes, putting this group at higher risk of type 2 diabetes and heart disease.

Since we know that certain habits that contribute to these risk factors, such as a sedentary lifestyle and a poor diet, develop early in life, this is a very disturbing statistic. Of all the Americans who have prediabetes, only 1 in 10 knows that he or she has it.

Many people mistakenly think that mild elevations in blood pressure don't affect them, but since our hearts beat on average 100,000 times per day, even small elevations in blood pressure are multiplied throughout the day and have a huge effect.

Think of your heart as a muscle lifting weights every time it pumps. If it has to pump out blood against higher pressure, your heart works harder and the muscle gets thicker. On routine heart tests of young adults, doctors are finding increased thickness of the heart walls and of heart mass. These are predictors for future heart events that can cause major damage, like heart attack and stroke.

Higher rates of depression and suicide And the research shows that it's not just because depression tends to spike in younger adults and be less prevalent in older age. It also can't be completely explained by the fact that younger generations are more likely to talk about mental illness and seek treatment.

Researchers don't know why mental health is declining among younger people. But some evidence points to contributing factors such as:

- **Internet use and online bullying.** They've both been associated with depression, self-harm, and suicidal thoughts and behaviors.
- **Less sleep.** Some studies have shown that young adults are sleeping fewer hours per night. And sleep disturbance has been linked to poor mental health and suicidal behaviors. On the other hand, an increase in depression and other mental illnesses could be what's causing young adults to get less sleep.

More signs of stress Millennials seem to be just as stressed as Generation X before them, and significantly more stressed than the baby boomers. In a study conducted by the American Psychological Association, millennials were more likely than older generations to say that their stress had increased in the last year. And over half of millennials reported having lain awake at night in the past month because of stress. Fewer people from older generations reported having that problem. Whether this is a function of age or a sign of the times is unclear.

These trends might seem grim. But the good news is that you can make a big impact on your health and your risk of disease through small, manageable actions you take every day. It's just a matter of figuring out what works for you to make healthy habits stick.

KNOW YOUR BRAIN

To get new healthy habits to stick, research shows that our brains need more than logical arguments. And they even need more than repetition. Our brains need rewards.

Why? Our brains rely on ingrained habits for everything from how we eat to how we respond to criticism. In fact, at least half of what we do is habitual — meaning that how we live our daily lives is governed just as much by habit as it is by thought.

There's a reason for this. Our brains, similar to the rest of our bodies, want to be efficient and conserve energy. In other words, our brains want to do as little work as possible. Repetitive, automated tasks give the brain less work to do. That means that even if some of our habits are hurting us, our brains resist changing them. Ideas of what we *should* do for our long-term health usually just aren't strong enough to battle with that habit-forming part of the brain. Our brains need more than just good intentions to change established patterns.

The good news is that research shows lasting change is totally possible. And starting the process of forming healthy habits and slowly modifying unhealthy ones when you're younger will make those healthy choices easier to sustain as you age.

But to set new habits you'll need frequent, immediate rewards to trigger production of the neurotransmitter dopamine, stimulating your brain to lay down new habit memory. For a new habit to stick, it needs to make sense in your life and give you enough positive feeling to keep coming back for more.

Chapter 4 is all about setting yourself up for successful change and contains extensive information on how to change. But the key idea is to set small goals you know you can achieve. Goals that are too big often lead to failure. Failure tells your brain, don't repeat that experience.

So instead of vowing to go to the gym every day for an hour, for example, go once a week for 15 minutes. Or if that's too much, just get ready for the gym once a week, even if you don't go. Focus on achieving that initial success, which will then allow your brain to feel the reward and build on it.

ENJOY WHAT YOU DO

For many of us, thinking about our health can bring up feelings of guilt and shame. Such feelings could be about our bodies and how we look, or about habits we know might hurt us in the long term but help us cope in the here and now. For some, focusing on "being healthy" can trigger feelings

AT LEAST HALF OF WHAT WE DO IS HABITUAL. OUR DAILY LIVES ARE GOVERNED JUST AS MUCH BY HABIT AS BY THOUGHT.

of shame or failure when well-intentioned plans fall through. Or for some it can lead to obsessive, unsustainable rounds of dieting and exercise. Such thinking often involves an all-or-nothing approach.

Healthy habits shouldn't be a form of self-punishment. They should make you feel good. Research shows that self-compassion is significantly more effective than self-blame or shame when it comes to sticking with habits over time.

Don't keep trying to develop a healthy habit that you don't like or enjoy. It is doomed to fail. Instead, search for a variation of that habit or aspiration that fits you. For example, your friend has taken up jogging and you can see the benefits that have resulted — your friend is becoming fit and trim and has more energy. Being fit and trim and having more energy are things you aspire to, as well. So you decide to take up jogging. The only problem is that you hate jogging and just can't get into it, even after multiple attempts.

But wait. There are other ways to achieve your aspirations. First, think of physical ac-tivities that you like to do and that fit into your lifestyle and capabilities. Then narrow this list down to those that are easy for you to do. Finally, pick one that you can easily link to an existing part of your routine. The easier and more enjoyable you make it, the less friction there will be around developing the new habit, and the more successful you'll be.

IF NOT FOR YOURSELF, THEN FOR THE EARTH

My wife, Linda, and I have three children who are all millennials in their late 20s and early 30s. I've talked to them about how important what they eat is when it comes to lowering their chance of disease. They've basically said, "Why should we worry about that when we're young, healthy and many years away from developing any kind of disease?" But when I told them that eating less red meat and dairy could bring their carbon footprint down by 70%, their perspective changed. The benefits suddenly seemed more immediate.

If you're like many millennials, you have climate change and the health of the Earth

MULTITASKING HABITS

Millennials love to get things done. That's why they're so productive. With that in mind, here are some ways to accomplish multiple health goals in one step.

Moving for your mind Exercise has immediate mental health benefits:

- It lowers stress and anxiety immediately. It's like taking an aspirin for a head-ache. Even a 10-minute walk when you're feeling really anxious can provide hours of relief.
- It improves cognitive function. Exercise has been shown to improve memory, attention and executive-control processes (such as the ability to plan and organize, as well as control emotions).
- It can help you sleep better tonight. Quality sleep is an important contributor to mental health.

In the long term, regular exercise can lower your risk of depression and anxiety. It can also improve symptoms if you live with mental illness already. People who get regular exercise also tend to have better mental processing speed, memory and decision-making skills.

Even small amounts of regular exercise — as little as 10 minutes three times a week — can lower your risk of heart disease, high blood pressure, type 2 diabetes, many cancers, dementia, and more. The benefits are there regardless of body size or shape.

Meditating for your body Evidence shows that meditation can improve symptoms of depression and anxiety, as well as help with psychological distress and anger or hostility. But because of the mind-body connection, meditation can have real effects on physical health too. It's been shown to:

- Improve sleep quality, even among people with insomnia
- Lower blood pressure in people who are at higher risk of developing high blood pressure
- Improve pain and quality of life in people with irritable bowel syndrome (IBS)
- Help some people with chronic pain

on the brain. Luckily, habits that are good for you can also bring down your carbon footprint.

Researchers have studied the relationship between diets that are healthy for people and diets that are healthy for the Earth. And the happy results are that the two often go together.

Bad news first: On a global scale, food production is one of the largest contributors to climate change. Food production and agriculture contribute up to 30% of all greenhouse gas emissions, occupy 40% of the available land on Earth, and use 70% of all available fresh water. And scientific modeling predicts that unless dietary patterns change, by 2050 we will likely see an 80%

EVERYDAY WAYS TO PRACTICE MEDITATION

Don't let the thought of meditating the "right" way add to your stress. You can certainly attend special meditation centers or group classes led by trained instructors. But you can also practice meditation easily on your own. All you really need is a few minutes of quality time. Here are some ways to try:

- **Breathe deeply.** This technique is good for beginners because breathing is a natural function. Focus all your attention on your breathing. Concentrate on feeling and listening as you inhale and exhale through your nostrils. Breathe deeply and slowly.
- **Scan your body.** Become aware of your body's various sensations, whether that's pain, tension, warmth or relaxation. Combine body scanning with breathing exercises, and imagine breathing heat or relaxation into and out of different parts of your body.
- **Repeat a mantra.** A common example of a mantra is the om chant of Hinduism. You can also create your own mantra, whether it's a favorite word, phrase or prayer that you repeat over and over.
- **Walk and meditate.** Combining a walk with meditation is an efficient and healthy way to relax. Slow down your walking pace so that you can focus on lifting each foot, moving your leg forward and placing your foot on the ground.
- **Engage in prayer.** Prayer is the best known and most widely practiced example of meditation. Spoken and written prayers are found in most faith traditions. You can pray using your own words or read prayers written by others.

increase in agricultural greenhouse gas emissions and global land clearing.

The good news is that dietary changes that are better for people's health tend to line up with the kinds of changes that would reduce greenhouse gas emissions and mitigate the effects of climate change.

The diets that use more land and water and produce more greenhouse gases tend to be high in added sugar, saturated fats, processed foods and red meat. And animal products account for 70% of greenhouse gas emissions in the diets of people in high-income nations like the United States.

Moving toward a diet that's higher in whole, plant-based foods like fruits, veggies, nuts, seeds and whole grains and lower in processed and animal-based foods can decrease your health risks while also reducing your carbon footprint.

Millennials are now the largest living generation in the U.S. That gives this generation power to change the kinds of foods that are most in demand and the ways those foods are produced.

Other healthy habits that help the earth:

- **Commuting green.** Biking, walking or taking public transit to get from place to place makes your days more active and means you're burning fewer fossil fuels.
- **Shopping local.** Spending your food money at the local farmers market means you're more likely to buy whole, plant-based foods with less packaging and less energy needed to transport the foods. Plus, local, small-scale food producers are more likely to use organic practices that are good for the land. Some local farmers are flash freezing their produce and making it available for purchase in the nonharvest months.
- **Growing your own food.** Gardening in your backyard or at a community garden can produce healthy food and keep you active. It can also contribute to more green space around you and provide habitat for animals and pollinators. To get started, try something simple such as a tomato plant, which is the vegetable most frequently grown at home.

MONEY AND YOUR HEALTH

Let's be real. Healthy living isn't just a matter of willpower. It's easier to make choices that are good for your health when you have more money, time and access to resources. The financial barriers to making healthy choices aren't excuses. They're a reality.

Many millennials were trying to start their careers during the Great Recession of 2007-2009, and lack of job opportunities during that time had lasting effects for some. And while they are the most educated generation yet, real wages for millennials have stayed stagnant compared with wages of baby boomers at the same age. Add to that student debt and the rising costs of housing and health care, and many millennials are short on disposable income.

And making healthy choices can be costly. Healthy foods can be more expensive than processed convenience foods. Gym memberships can be expensive. Cooking healthy meals, exercising regularly and taking steps to manage stress all take time, which is harder to come by if you're working long hours or multiple jobs on top of all the other things in life.

But whatever your circumstances, there are steps you can take to improve your health, and investing time and money in healthy living when you're young could pay off financially in the long run. Health care is expensive, and the Centers for Medicare and Medicaid Services projects that the cost of health care services will continue to rise between 2018 and 2027.

The key is to take small steps that you can afford and that make sense in your life. Those small things can add up to make a big difference in your health, and they don't have to cost too much.

Small, cheap habits with big health payoffs:

- **Move more during the day.** Physical activity is good for you, even if it's in small doses. No time or money for a run to the gym? Build activity into your day. Take the stairs. Walk while you're talking on the phone. Go for a 10-minute run, or run for two minutes if you don't have time for 10. Also, try to move every hour — even walking to speak with a colleague instead of making a call or sending an email is helpful. Why is even a small effort like this beneficial? Because that's

what your body is programmed to do. People never used to sit around all day a million years ago. They had to get up and move frequently to survive the day.

- **Cut back on meat.** Evidence shows that a diet that's packed with plants more than with animal products tends to be healthier and decrease health risks. And meat can take up a big part of your food budget. Switching out meat for inexpensive canned or frozen beans and legumes in some of your meals could save you money and bring more plants into your diet.
- **Go for frozen produce.** Fruits and vegetables that have been flash frozen preserve almost all of their nutrients. And they tend to be less expensive than fresh produce. They're also convenient to store and easy to add to a meal.
- **Make social time active.** Social life in your 20s and 30s can be heavy on eating out and getting drinks. Getting in the habit of asking friends to go for walks, go dancing, go bowling or play an active game can give you two benefits at once: social time and physical activity. And you spend less money on getting drinks and eating out.

RETHINKING FAMILY HISTORY

Family health history can feel heavy. If someone in your family has had heart disease, diabetes, cancer, or another chronic or serious disease, you probably know that your risk of getting the same disease may be higher than someone without a family history of these conditions.

It's true that for some diseases, genetic factors can play a big role. But for many diseases and health conditions, the way you live every day has far more to do with your risk than your genes.

Research shows that about 75% of strokes can be prevented by having a healthy lifestyle. And lifestyle and environmental factors play a role in about half of all cancer cases.

While it's true that you're never too old to make healthy changes that can make a real difference, it's also true that making needed changes earlier in life can yield higher rewards.

A study that followed over 3,000 participants for 20 years, from their mid-20s to their mid-40s, showed that starting and staying with healthy habits in early adulthood can significantly lower your risk of

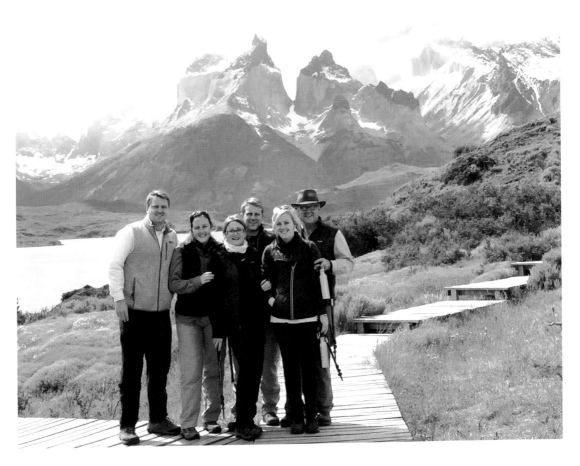

We combined outside exercise and fun on a family vacation to Patagonia, Chile, in 2016 at the Torres del Paine National Park.

3 TIPS FOR MILLENNIAL PARENTS

You can do a lot for your kids' health just by being a good example.

1. **Model healthy living and habits.** Children learn best by example. Millennials are the largest demographic group now and are in the prime child-raising years. Children establish many of their eating habits by age 12 and activity habits at a somewhat younger age. Engage your children in healthy eating and exercise with activities centered around shopping for food and preparing it, walks in the local park, and going to playgrounds. When children have fun doing these activities, it leaves a permanent happy memory that guides them toward healthy decisions when they're on their own. What they learn to do early in life sets their nutrition and exercise patterns for the next 50-plus years.

2. **Lead by example when it comes to digital screen time.** Balance is key. Smartphones, computers and the internet are all necessary, but be an example to your children on how to manage screens and screen time. Spend time with them without a screen, too. It reminds them of how important they are to you.

3. **Show kids how to make a positive change.** Find a couple of habits that you'd like to improve and make a tiny change now. Link it to something that you do frequently, make it enjoyable and encourage your children to join in. Maybe your family loves cheese. Instead of giving up cheese altogether, add slices of apple or pear to go with it. Slice the cheese a little thinner — you'll still get the great flavor. This gives you an extra serving of fruit for the day and can become a healthy, fun habit over time.

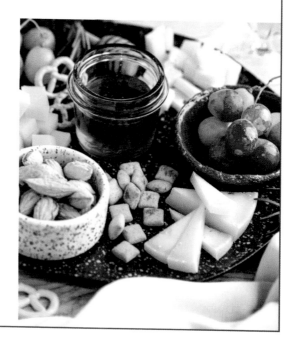

heart disease later in life, even if someone in your family has had it.

So for many of us, what we have to confront is less about the genetic risks we inherit and more about the habits we learned from our families. Most people have some family patterns and habits they'd like to keep and carry on and others they'd like to put to rest.

Parents and guardians play a huge role in teaching kids behaviors and attitudes around food, exercise, sleep, stress and so much more. Examining what you learned from your own upbringing and knowing what you want for your own children can help empower you to set your own goals and habits even if they're new and unfamiliar.

If you have access to your family history, talk to your doctor about what that history means for you. What does a grandmother having breast cancer mean for your risk? What about a parent living with a heart condition? And what are the most important lifestyle factors that could bring down your risk of the diseases in your family history?

If you're a parent or you want to be one, know that by making healthy changes, you're providing a positive example for your kids that could change the health trajectory of their lives.

FINDING WHAT WORKS FOR YOU

There isn't one right way to eat, exercise, stay motivated or care for yourself. In the rest of this book, you'll find more information about the daily habits known to be the most beneficial at lowering your risk of disease. How you absorb that information and what changes you decide to make are going to be part of your own personal journey.

The keys to long-term healthy habits: Having the information you need to make informed choices, finding motivators and strategies for change that are physically and mentally healthy for you, and being kind to yourself throughout the process.

IT'S NEVER TOO LATE TO MAKE LIFE BETTER.

CHAPTER 6

For baby boomers

What about baby boomers? Is it too late to turn things around? As you enter your 60s and 70s, it's tempting to think that your best years are behind you.

You may be feeling some new aches and pains. Maybe your cholesterol is higher than you'd like, your waistline is growing or that stiffness in your fingers is becoming more persistent.

You might be wishing you had taken better care of yourself in past years. Maybe, looking back, you wish you'd eaten a little more salad than steak. Or gotten more sleep. Or taken your running shoes out more times.

But be gentle with yourself. Regret doesn't improve your health. Action does. And make no mistake: It's never too late to make choices that will improve your health.

Making healthy changes now — even if you're over 65 — can help you feel as good as you did in your 40s and 50s. Even small changes, like taking one more bite of a healthy food or doing three minutes of vigorous exercise, can make a difference in your daily life and improve your health span.

DISEASES OF LONG LIFE

As many people enter their 60s and 70s, they begin to grow more concerned about diseases typically associated with aging, like dementia and cancer. They watch for worrisome signs, like unusual new pains or memory lapses, and fear that these conditions have caught up with them. Sometimes they become so preoccupied with these health concerns that they neglect more-pressing health matters.

It's true that the risk of dementia and some cancers do rise with age. But today's baby boomers are much more likely to have another condition: heart disease.

Why is this?

Compared with people of similar age spans, baby boomers are more likely than the previous generation to make choices that lead to heart disease. They get significantly less physical activity than their parents did. They are more likely to be overweight or obese. They're also more likely to have high cholesterol, diabetes and high blood pressure.

Changes that occur more commonly with age also can increase the risk of heart disease. For instance, your large arteries may stiffen (arteriosclerosis), and yearslong plaque buildup can cause the walls of arteries to narrow (atherosclerosis). Age-related changes in your heart may result in an irregular heartbeat (arrhythmia), stiff valves and heart chambers that grow in size.

The resulting heart disease can significantly affect people's lives. It limits activity, leads to medical interventions and decreases quality of life for millions of people every year. And it remains the most common cause of death in older adults.

That doesn't mean that cancer, dementia and diabetes aren't concerns as you age.

Cancer follows heart disease as the second leading cause of death in older adults. And age is the most important risk factor. Nearly 50% of new cancer cases are found in people who are between the ages of 65 and 84.

Rates of dementia, a condition that affects memory, thinking and social abilities, increase with age as well. And the incidence is growing alongside the growth in life span. In fact, some research suggests that dementia may affect more than 150 million people worldwide by 2050 — up from about 50 million in 2019.

Risk of type 2 diabetes, a condition that affects how the body uses blood sugar and can have many complications, also increases with age. And, as with dementia, cases of diabetes are on the rise overall — due in large part to factors that can be controlled, like inactivity, poor diet and obesity. Research shows that by 2050, diabetes may affect around a third of adults in the U.S., and I have absolutely no doubt that will happen.

All of these diseases of a long life — heart disease, cancer, dementia, diabetes and others — are worth your attention. And, more importantly, your action. Because you do have the power to prevent or slow them.

SLOWING THE HANDS OF TIME

It's never too late to make a change. And when it comes to improving your health — and your health span — there's no time like the present.

Don't let excuses hold you back. It doesn't matter if you're closer to 75 than 65. Or if

THE EFFECTS OF AGING

It's true that as we age, our bodies get a little worn. They become more fragile and more susceptible to injury and chronic illness. For example, our blood vessels tend to get stiffer, causing our hearts to work harder to pump blood at an appropriate rate. Our heart muscles change to adjust to the increased workload, raising the risk of high blood pressure and other heart problems.

Our bones tend to shrink in size and density, making them weaker and more susceptible to fracture. Muscles generally lose some of their strength, endurance and flexibility. Our skin gets wrinkly and less elastic. Our brains undergo changes that have minor effects on memory and thinking skills. We may forget familiar names or words or find it hard to multitask.

But changes that come with age are not the same as those that occur with chronic illness. Aging may make us more vulnerable to disease, but it doesn't cause it. Our actions at any age can help. Remember, nothing we do to improve our health is ever too little, and it's never too late, no matter when we start. We can make choices that improve our ability to maintain an active life, do the things we enjoy and spend time with those we love.

you haven't exercised in 20 years — or longer. Or if you can't remember the last time you ate a vegetable that wasn't deep-fried.

If you commit to eating healthy foods and getting more physical activity now, you can still lower your risk of heart disease, cancer, dementia and other chronic conditions. You'll strengthen muscles and bones, reduce your risk of injury, and move more easily in your daily life. You'll sleep better and improve your mental function. You'll boost your mood and have more energy.

In short, you will slow the aging process and increase your health span. Making healthy choices truly does slow the hands of time. Research has shown that even after age 65, an improved diet and physical activity can slow the aging process. For every year that you live, the things we typically think of as "aging" — such as decreased mental sharpness and memory, decreased walking speed, and increased body aches — are slowed by 25% with changes in diet and regular physical activity. Another way to think of this that may motivate you is that small changes in your diet and physical activity can reduce your aging. By how much? As you'll read later, these changes allow you to live another year but only age 9 months!

So, what does moving more and eating better after age 65 look like? What exactly do you need to do to achieve these benefits?

For starters, if you smoke, it's not too late to stop. You'll reduce your risk of dozens of diseases — including heart disease and 12 different kinds of cancer. Research shows that quitting smoking can actually increase your life expectancy up to 10 years. If you drink too much alcohol, slow down to a drink a day or quit altogether.

Not sleeping well? Practice good sleep hygiene and talk to your doctor about options that can help. Practice stress-reducing techniques and connect with friends and family. Those measures alone will improve your quality of life at any age.

However, two of the most powerful actions to improve your daily life and your health span are increasing your physical activity and changing your diet.

Physical activity

As a child, you were probably pretty physically active — running and playing and taking part in many activities. Even if you continued to stay vigorously active for only 10 minutes three times a week as you jour-

neyed through adulthood, you've already done a tremendous amount to help prevent health problems that can occur over time. And I know most of you are thinking, "I've done that." Maybe you have, but currently only 1 in 5 adults in the U.S. is doing so.

Most of us don't stay as active as we were when we were children, or even as active as we were in our 20s and 30s. Hours of sitting at a desk or in a recliner watching TV replace our once busy lifestyle. Many of us are now faced with fixing health issues caused by inactivity — like high blood pressure, heart disease and obesity.

But it's never too late to get moving. Even small improvements can significantly affect your health. Get started with this advice:

- **Ease in.** Slow and steady wins this race. If you've been sedentary, start with some stretches and a walk down your street. Then increase your activity as you're able.
- **Focus on activity instead of exercise.** Going on a bike ride, gardening, fishing, golfing, dancing, playing pickleball and doing yoga in your living room all count.
- **Work it into your routine.** Do some stretches or lift hand weights while watching TV. Or, instead of meeting a friend for coffee, go for a walk together.
- **Don't overdo it.** If using weights, start with 1 or 2 pounds. If using resistance bands, start with the most flexible band and work your way up.
- **Get social.** Exercising with a friend can be a great motivator — and more fun. Ask friends or family to go on bike rides

or take yoga classes with you. Studies have shown that social activities, like tennis, lead to greater health benefits than solo activities like running or going to the gym alone (see pages 194 and 195).

- **Work with what you've got.** Don't let disabilities or medical conditions keep you from being active. For instance, swimming may be an option for those who have difficulty walking. And exercise can actually decrease your arthritis pain.
- **Talk to your doctor or health care provider.** Make sure you're healthy enough for the activities you want to do. Your care provider can offer advice and recommend an exercise program that works for you.

Healthy diet

Diet is more than getting three square meals a day. It's the best medicine you can take — a daily dose of prevention to help optimize your health. In fact, researchers have found that seniors who eat a healthy diet may have longer lives.

The Mediterranean diet has been shown to have a range of health benefits. With its focus on fruits, vegetables, beans and legumes, whole grains, healthy oils, and fish, it offers vital nutrition for both body and mind.

In a study of more than 2,000 people age 60 and older, those who more closely followed a Mediterranean diet had less "functional deterioration." In other words, their memory and other mental functions, like focus and attention, were better maintained over the course of the study. In fact, for every one chronological year, those who followed a Mediterranean diet had only aged the equivalent of nine months. Reduced consumption of red or processed meat and sugar-sweetened beverages, and increased intake of fish were the main contributors to the difference between groups.

In one study of 5,000 people age 65 and older, those who closely followed a Mediterranean diet had better heart health — and their risk of death from all causes was reduced.

The Mediterranean diet can also be a powerful prevention tool against other health concerns commonly faced in the final decades of life. It's associated with a reduced risk of cancer, diabetes, dementia, Parkinson's disease, high blood pressure and macular degeneration. It helps reduce arthritis pain, improve cholesterol levels and aids in weight loss.

Combine this diet with regular physical activity and you have a winning retirement plan. A plan that you can take into a long, active and full future.

CHANGING YOUR LIFESTYLE IMPROVES YOUR BRAIN

Researchers wanted to determine whether exercise and diet could help people improve their ability to plan, focus, learn new things and juggle multiple tasks (executive functions), even once these skills had begun to deteriorate slightly.

They studied a group of adults over age 55 who had some signs of impairment but not dementia, who were at risk of coronary artery disease, and who were fairly sedentary. The study lasted six months. Participants were split up into four treatment groups:

1. The first group engaged in aerobic exercise three times a week. The exercise routine consisted of 10 minutes of warm-up exercises followed by 35 minutes of continuous walking or stationary cycling. Participants were encouraged to follow their usual diets.

2. Participants in the second group modified their diets to follow the guidelines of the Dietary Approaches to Stop Hypertension (DASH) diet. The DASH diet is similar to the Mediterranean diet but with an added focus on reducing salt. These participants met regularly with a nutrition specialist and were told not to exercise.

3. The third group received instructions on incorporating aerobic exercise and the DASH diet into their lives, as detailed above.

4. The fourth group received regular phone calls from a health educator on heart disease-related topics. These participants maintained their usual dietary and exercise habits.

The researchers measured the participants' executive functions before and after the trial. They found that increasing aerobic exercise and switching to the DASH diet did indeed improve executive functioning after the trial period of six months. As you can see from the chart, the most benefit came when exercise and diet changes were combined.

When you compare the scores of those who modified their diet and exercise habits with those who maintained their usual routine, you can see what a big difference it made.

BRAIN FUNCTION IMPROVES QUICKLY
6 MONTHS

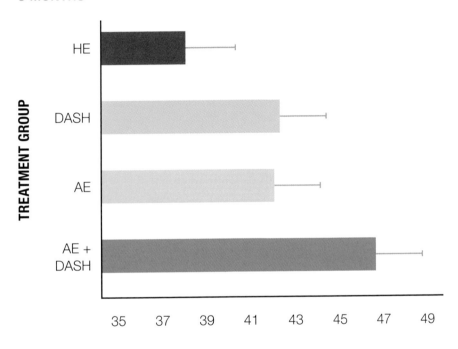

TREATMENT GROUP

HE

DASH

AE

AE + DASH

35   37   39   41   43   45   47   49

EXECUTIVE FUNCTIONS SCORE

HE = Health education

DASH = Dietary Approach to Stop Hypertension

AE = Aerobic exercise

Based on Neurology. 2019;92:e212.

THE POWER OF PURPOSE

For many people today, the retirement years are a long-awaited prize, the payoff for years of hard work. You may have pictured a life of leisure filled with hobbies and travel, golfing, and time spent with family and friends. And then, suddenly, you're facing these years faster than you imagined. So fast that you may find yourself thinking: "Now what?"

You may have difficulty creating an identity outside of your career. You may be surprised to find that you miss the structure of a regular workday and the community it can bring. You may worry that stepping away from your job also means stepping away from the purpose and meaning you found there.

These are common feelings. But as my physician father — who died at 91, two weeks after seeing his last patient — told me many times, "You have to retire *to* something, not *from* something." It's important to think of retirement as moving to a full, new life of promise, adventure and purpose.

In retirement, you're given the opportunity to pursue activities that fill your soul instead of your timecard. And you're given the freedom to take action — whether that means building meaningful relationships, exploring your creativity or diving deeper into an interest you've always had.

Maybe you find meaning in helping an older neighbor take care of her house or in babysit-

ting a grandchild. Maybe you mentor an up-and-comer or volunteer with an organization you love. Whatever it is, find that purpose in your life. Find your "why" — why do you want to wake up tomorrow, and what do you want to do with every new day?

This is your time to focus on what's truly important to you — and how you're going to make the most of this next chapter of your life. After I had my second cancer, I found great comfort in focusing on every day as if it might be my last. Sometimes I would think, "What if I were on a plane that was going to crash, how would I focus my last moments?" Then I would do just that.

LIVING YOUR BEST LIFE

Knowing what you want out of life can be a great motivator. So once you understand your meaning and purpose, use that as inspiration to live your best life.

Here's one way to think about it: In your 20s, you want to conquer the world. In your 30s and 40s, you start realizing you probably aren't going to. And in your 50s, 60s and beyond, you accept who you are, recognize your purpose, and enjoy some of your best years of happiness, well-being and freedom from worry. That's why 60-and 70-year-olds are some of the happiest people on the planet.

More than any other time in your life, your senior years are when you're more likely to have a solid sense of who you are, how you want to spend your time and what really matters to you. For many, this is a time of gratitude, optimism and happiness — a combination that pays off in more than just warm, fuzzy feelings. It actually improves your health and well-being. Here's what the research says about the concrete benefits of these three overlapping traits.

Gratitude Everyone feels thankful at times. You receive a gift or need help with something and you feel grateful to the person who thought of you or came to your aid. But gratitude can be inspired by more than just tangible or immediate benefits. You might be thankful for a loving family or a rewarding job. You might feel awed and

HOW TO FIND YOUR 'WHY'

Not sure what your why in life is?

You're not alone. Many older adults wrestle with finding meaning as they transition into older adulthood and the final decades of their lives. But uncovering your purpose is a worthwhile exercise that can significantly affect your happiness, health and well-being.

Ask yourself the following questions to help uncover the purpose in your life — and the best places to focus your energy:

- What activities make me feel excited, fulfilled or rewarded?
- When do I feel like the best version of me?
- What are my natural gifts, talents and abilities?
- How do I best help others?
- What three (or five or seven) ideas, actions or events are most important to me?
- What have I always wanted to try?
- What activities do I most look forward to each day, week or month?
- What have I been putting off until I have more time?
- What relationships are most important to me?
- Are there relationships that I'd like to make stronger or invest more time in?
- What do I want my days to look like? What about my weeks and years?
- Does it feel like something is missing from my life? What is it?
- If I could do anything, what would it be?

grateful when surrounded by natural beauty. Or you might experience a more esoteric appreciation of life if you narrowly escape a dangerous situation.

However, transient moments of thankfulness aren't enough to explain the wider concept of gratitude. Gratitude, especially as it correlates to a higher sense of well-being, is a way of being that habitually focuses on noticing and appreciating the positive aspects of life. It's being thankful for the people and experiences that make up your life.

People who score high on measures of gratitude understand that they have much to be thankful for. They reflect on how fortunate they are to have basic things such as food, clothing and shelter. They realize that things could be worse, that life is short and that it's important to enjoy life as it is.

Practicing gratitude doesn't mean giving up ambitions and goals. It means you're able to be content in the moment even as you pursue long-term plans. A grateful approach enables you to be happy despite the imperfections of life.

Gratitude does more than just create positive feelings. In surveys, a disposition toward thankfulness predicted a decreased risk of mental health disorders. It also helped people overcome trauma. A number of studies support a link between gratitude and being in a good mood and feeling happier and more satisfied with life. Gratitude has also been linked to self-acceptance, independence from peer pressure, personal growth, and a sense of purpose and control over your circumstances.

One study even found that higher levels of gratitude resulted in better sleep. Results

HOW TO PRACTICE GRATITUDE

Do you want to spend more time practicing gratitude but aren't sure how to begin? Consider these ideas:

- Keep a gratitude journal, writing down the things you're grateful for each day.
- Think about the people in your life who you're grateful for before getting out of bed in the morning.
- Write a letter to a loved one, expressing your appreciation for them.
- Meditate on or pray for the things you're grateful for before going to sleep at night.
- Write thank-you notes for the gifts in your life.

showed that grateful people sleep better because they worry less and have fewer negative thoughts before falling asleep. They also tend to focus on positive things before falling asleep, which protects the quality of their rest.

Optimism Optimism is that hopeful or confident feeling that things are going to work out for the better. It's a positive outlook that actually doubles as a stress reliever.

Research shows that optimistic people have a reduced risk of heart disease and heart attack. In one study, more than 7,000 people were taught positive thinking along with gratitude practices. At the end of the five-year study, their chance of heart attack had been lowered by 25%.

What was the positive thinking the participants were doing? Every morning when they woke up or every evening when they went to bed, they thought of three things they were thankful for that day. These could've been small things, inconsequential to others, but nonetheless worthy of gratitude. After a few years, heart attacks decreased, plus overall happiness and outlook on life improved.

Happiness Happiness is the feeling you get when you enjoy life and feel hopeful for the future. It's joy, positivity and the feeling that your life has meaning. People are often happier and more fulfilled at retirement age than in any other decade of life — in part because they're more confident, they know what matters most to them and they act on

it. They may finally have time to do what they want to do, whether that's pursuing long-held dreams, traveling or spending time with loved ones.

Research shows that this increase in happiness does more than boost emotional and mental health. It may also lead to a longer life. In one study, happy older people (age 60 and above) lived longer than unhappy older people. In fact, the likelihood of dying of any cause was 19% lower for the happy people studied.

None of us is going to check out of this world alive — but if you live with purpose and meaning and practice gratitude, optimism and happiness, you're going to live your fullest and most rewarding life.

YOUR BODY'S ABILITY TO FIGHT INFECTION DEPENDS MORE ON YOUR LIFESTYLE THAN YOU THINK.

CHAPTER 7

Boosting the immune system

In early 2020, life as most of the world knew it came to a screeching halt. That's when a previously unknown virus began spreading like wildfire, forcing businesses, office buildings, schools, stores, gyms, places of worship, restaurants, movie theaters and other public gathering places to shut their doors.

For our part, those of us who could hunkered down in our homes, hoping that avoiding mingling with others would help minimize transmission of the the virus and all of its possible complications.

The virus is now commonly known around the world as the coronavirus. The disease it causes is called coronavirus disease 2019 (COVID-19). In March 2020, the World Health Organization (WHO) declared the COVID-19 outbreak a global pandemic.

The pandemic impacted our lives in ways we couldn't have imagined. Yet it also told the same old story: We know our health impacts our longevity and quality of life, but we struggle to do the things that will boost our immune systems and help us live younger longer.

A NEW VIRUS COLLIDES WITH LONG-STANDING DISEASES

Although our knowledge of the virus and how it spread seemed to change by the hour, one fact remained the same: Illness can and did strike all sorts of people, but the vast majority who developed a severe case of COVID-19 had preexisting health problems. Those at higher risk had conditions such as obesity, high blood pressure, diabetes, heart disease, and a history of stroke or smoking.

Drawing on a database of around 500,000 people in the United Kingdom, scientists analyzed characteristics of those who tested positive for COVID-19 in 2020. Those with two or more long-term conditions had almost a 50% higher risk of COVID-19 infection. Two or more cardiometabolic conditions increased risk by 75%. Cardiometabolic diseases include long-term chronic conditions that affect the heart or blood vessels, or metabolism, such as obesity or kidney disease. Those taking 10 or more medicines had a 250% greater risk.

Chances of getting COVID-19 are higher when there's an underlying cardiometabolic disease, and subsequent chances of being placed on a respirator (intubated) or dying are also higher. In the study, those with underlying cardiometabolic conditions were almost 350% more likely to require intubation or die of COVID-19 than people who had COVID-19 but were otherwise healthy.

Change is hard

As discussed in previous chapters, small changes in everyday habits, such as eating one less bite of red meat or taking the stairs whenever you can, are important ways to help prevent these long-term chronic illnesses from developing.

These same healthy habits — as well as other habits such as washing hands and wearing a mask in public — can help prevent communicable diseases like COVID-19 by protecting our overall health and boosting our immune systems. And if an infection does occur, it's likely to be much less severe than if we were already in poor health.

Still, even in the face of an acute pandemic such as COVID-19, people had difficulty making changes, even when these changes were clearly and immediately beneficial to their health. Another recent study looking at prevention behaviors found that people with cardiometabolic diseases were least likely to practice "COVID healthy behaviors" in eight of 10 categories. The categories were the ones we heard about every day, such as wearing a mask, washing hands, social distancing, avoiding crowds and staying home when sick. It really points out how hard it is for humans to change habits, even when the consequences are two weeks away, not two decades.

If the possibility of catching a potentially fatal viral infection doesn't make us want to be healthier, then what does motivate us? I think part of the answer is that change is difficult when the desire for it doesn't come from within. As a doctor, I can advise my patients and you, my readers, about the risks and benefits of our lifestyles, but I cannot make you change your habits. Only you can do that. Only you can determine your own "why," your individual reason for striving for better health.

A double-edged sword

There's no doubt that in the COVID-19 example, prevention was a double-edged

RISK OF GETTING COVID-19

In this example, the risk of a healthy person getting COVID-19 is a factor of 1. That risk increases by 50% if you have two or more chronic conditions, 75% if these conditions involve your heart or metabolism, and 250% if you take 10 or more medications.

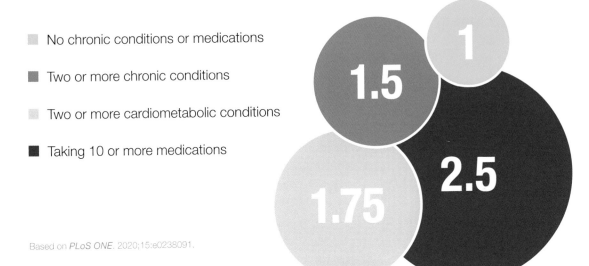

- No chronic conditions or medications
- Two or more chronic conditions
- Two or more cardiometabolic conditions
- Taking 10 or more medications

Based on *PLoS ONE*. 2020;15:e0238091.

---

sword. The best strategy to help contain the virus, a prolonged quarantine, also increased our sedentary behaviors. Many of us were stuck at home, sitting more and moving less (despite our best intentions), and sometimes eating more, too.

We were also stressed and anxious about things like job security, paying bills, grocery shopping and the impact of the virus on our kids' education. We struggled to sleep because of our worries, or smoked or drank more to combat stress. All of these habits, unfortunately, are what make us vulnerable to a wide variety of longterm illnesses.

But we also adjusted. We started taking more walks, working out at home and eating more intentionally. We remembered the importance of family and friends and cherished the sight of beloved faces on digital screens. We made do. We cried when we needed to and laughed whenever we could.

There will always be risk factors we can't change — genetics, sex, age or a global pandemic! But we can control other risk factors, such as what we put in our bodies and how much exercise and sleep we get. Prevention should be the cornerstone of medicine because it helps to prepare for the unexpected.

One thing I tell myself: "If you want to save a lot of lives, prevent disease; if you want to make a lot of money, treat disease." I'd much rather prevent disease. More often than not, though, health care providers end up seeing patients only after a problem has developed. COVID-19 highlighted why we need to be more proactive.

Understandably, a lot of time and effort was spent on finding a safe and effective vaccine following the emergence of COVID-19. But an important piece of the puzzle was inside of us all along.

IMMUNE SYSTEM BOOSTERS

We tend to take our immune systems for granted. But they work hard to keep us healthy. This complex system of cells is the body's primary defense system, constantly on the lookout for internal and external threats. To better understand how we can improve or boost the immune system, it helps to have a little background on how it works.

The immune system has two parts. There's the immune function that you're born with, called the innate immune system. The innate immune system is a general defense mechanism that protects you from the time your body is exposed to harmful germs till the time the second part of the immune response — the adaptive immune system — kicks in.

The adaptive immune system identifies and attacks specific germ invaders. It also remembers them, in case of a repeat exposure.

This allows your immune system to mount a more effective response the second time around. The process of inoculation develops when you get sick with a virus, or it can be developed intentionally with a vaccine.

When you get a flu shot, for example, you're essentially introducing your body to specific strains of the influenza virus that are too weak to cause illness but are recognizable enough to be encoded in your body's immune memory. When you subsequently encounter the flu virus in the community, your adaptive immune system recognizes it and goes to work to destroy it. It's estimated that there may be only a few thousand white blood cells in your body that are coded to recognize an invading virus. But once that invader is recognized, these cells replicate millions of times over to fight that specific infection.

Recognizing and destroying potentially dangerous invaders is only half of the job. The other part is being able to turn off that response quickly once the threat has been destroyed.

Immune responses take a lot of energy and result in inflammation — just think of the redness, swelling or pain you feel when you have a wound. It's a sign that your immune system is hard at work, and it's usually a good thing.

I say "usually" because, unfortunately, a sedentary lifestyle, unhealthy eating and excess fat create chronic low-level injuries that leave the immune system constantly switched on. Just think about a car idling. Leaving it running all the time would be bad for the car. The immune system is no different. Having it continuously on alert is bad for the body.

So what can we do to keep our immune systems healthy and strong?

Nutrition

The fuel you put into your body plays a critical role in how well your immune system works. But eating healthy foods and taking vitamins and other supplements after you're already sick doesn't provide the best response. Putting oil in your car after it's already overheated and broken down will prevent further damage to the engine, but it won't repair the harm that's already been done.

The key is prevention, so you have to make sure your body has what it needs to maintain a strong immune system. The word *nutrition* is derived from the Latin word *nutrix*, which is also the same root word that the

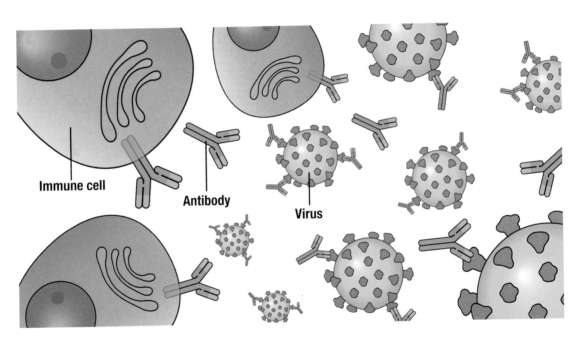

Immune cell **Antibody** **Virus**

Once you've been exposed to a germ invader such as a virus — whether through natural exposure or through a vaccine — your adaptive immune system kicks into gear. Adaptive immune cells produce antibodies that pinpoint and eliminate the invaders. The antibodies also remember the germs in case of a repeat exposure. When a repeat exposure occurs, your immune system mounts a more effective response than the first time around.

HEALTHY HABITS THAT BOOST YOUR IMMUNE SYSTEM

Healthy eating

Eating lots of fruits and vegetables provides antioxidants and anti-inflammatory nutrients that aid the immune system and help it fight infections.

Exercising

Regular moderate exercise increases the activity of virus-killing immune cells.

Managing stress and making connections

Calming activities and supportive relationships minimize stress, reduce cortisol production and enhance the immune system's function.

Getting enough sleep

Adequate sleep boosts the number of immune cells circulating in the body and improves infection outcomes.

term *nurse* is derived from. This is very appropriate and helps you understand that proper nutrition helps maintain your health, just like having a nurse at your side, tending to you and keeping you healthy.

A nutrition pattern that's rich in fruits and vegetables, such as the Mediterranean diet, serves up antioxidants and anti-inflammatory nutrients, such as beta carotene, vitamin C, vitamin E and polyphenols to promote healthy immune responses. Polyphenols are plant-based micronutrients that control how the immune system responds.

What we eat also helps the beneficial bacteria in our guts communicate with the immune system and with the lungs, allowing for a more effective response to foreign invaders, such as respiratory viruses. Any disruption to this delicate balance of bacteria, whether it's from an unhealthy diet or medication such as an antibiotic, can make you more susceptible to infections and complications.

Also, and equally if not more important, the Mediterranean diet, described in Chapter 8, has proved to be one of the most anti-inflammatory diets ever studied. Why is this helpful?

When we regularly eat foods that are pro-inflammatory, such as an excess of processed foods, they promote chronic inflammation in our bodies that requires our immune systems' attention. This constant inflammation requires our bodies to address the inflammation and heal it, which in turn diverts and lessens our immune systems' ability to recognize and fight other inflammatory processes such as an invading infection.

As a result, proper nutrition has dual benefits for our immune systems, both for what it does and for what it doesn't do. First, it allows the body to function better to fight infection. Second, it doesn't cause inflammation, which would further divert our immune systems' defenses.

We know from research on other diseases that certain vitamin deficiencies can lead to a tougher road to recovery for some people. For example, low levels of vitamin A may lead to complications if you contract measles, diarrheal disease, malaria or HIV/AIDS. In general, not consuming enough vitamins A, E, B-6 and B-12, along with zinc and selenium, have been linked in research to poorer recovery from a viral infection. Reduced levels of vitamin C, omega-3 fatty acids and iron also may negatively impact immune response.

There isn't definitive proof that supplementing with vitamins and minerals can ward off any particular virus. But eating nutritious foods as part of an overall healthy diet can help to optimize your immune system, setting you up for the best possible response.

Exercise

Exercise has been shown to give the immune system a boost by maximizing the body's ability to take in and efficiently use oxygen, among other things. Moderate exercise (where you can talk but not sing while exercising) is enough to increase the activity of virus-killing cells both in the short term and long term. This includes white blood cells and antibodies. Guidelines recommend at least 30 minutes daily, five times a week. But even 20 minutes daily can help quell inflammation and boost immunity, and exercise can be divided up during the day.

The best part about exercise is that it can be done at home, which, as we learned, is crucial when we're in the middle of a pandemic shutdown. Leg lunges, situps, squats and stair climbing are all easy exercises you can do at home.

Stress relief

During the COVID-19 pandemic, everyone has been feeling more stress than usual. Concern about the health of our loved ones, our jobs and our children's schooling combined with the inability to physically stay in touch with each other has been difficult. Such added stress increases production of the hormone cortisol in the body, which in turn can suppress the immune system.

Calming activities minimize stress, reduce cortisol production and enhance the immune system's function.

Practicing mindfulness and stepping away from what's causing anxiety can help us stay grounded. Exercises that have calming or meditative qualities, such as qi gong and yoga, also are beneficial and can easily be done at home. Video calls can help us stay connected to loved ones and reduce the stress of not being able to get together in person.

A few months into the pandemic, my wife and I hadn't been able to visit with our children, but we did talk with them frequently on the phone. My wife missed seeing them and was concerned whether they were staying healthy, eating well and being physically active.

Realizing that almost 90% of communication is nonverbal, we decided it would be good for us to set up some video calls with all of the family. It was therapeutic for both of us to see that the kids looked good and were surviving quite well.

Surprisingly, or maybe not, the benefit of the audiovisual interaction for our family was possibly even greater for our children than it was for us. For them, being able to see that their older parents were healthy and coping with the pandemic relieved a lot

THE IMPORTANCE OF THE FLU VACCINE

One of the best defenses against preventable, potentially dangerous complications of viruses such as the flu is getting vaccinated. This is particularly true if you have chronic heart disease, as you're more likely to have flu complications. Research has shown that in people with heart disease, flu vaccines can reduce the risk of events such as heart attacks, strokes and death from a cardiovascular event. Why? Because avoiding the flu and the resultant inflammatory response the body mounts reduces these cardiovascular events.

When you have an inflammatory reaction somewhere in the body, it affects the whole body. For example, having an event such as a bladder infection or even surgery increases your risk of a heart attack. This is due to the presence of inflamed white blood cells (and the compounds they secrete) circulating throughout the bloodstream. When these white blood cells come into contact with an artery in your heart that may already be inflamed from high blood pressure, high cholesterol or stress, the combination causes further inflammation in the artery. The increased inflammation can result in a tear in the lining of the blood vessel. This situation can lead to a local blood clot blocking the artery and causing a heart attack (see also the illustration on page 27).

of their stress. Stress reduction activities that involve others are beneficial to all parties.

Sleep

The interaction between the immune system and sleep is a two-way street. When your immune system response kicks in, it changes your sleep. You may find yourself sleeping longer, for example, as your immune system stages an attack against a virus.

On the flip side, when you don't get enough sleep, your immune system can be altered. When you're not sleeping well, you may notice that you get sick more easily. Getting adequate sleep can help support the way your immune system functions by increasing the number of immune cells circulating in your body.

Sleep has been associated with reduced infection risks, improved infection outcomes and better vaccination responses. Getting adequate sleep before receiving a vaccination can double the immune response in humans. Animal studies have shown that increasing the length of sleep positively affects infection outcomes.

Not getting enough sleep appears to be a trigger of low-grade inflammation and related diseases. Studies in humans on the relationship between sleep and infection link shorter sleep duration with increased risk of pneumonia and respiratory infections. The amount of sleep the immune system needs to function properly is very individual. But if suboptimal sleep is leaving you tired and run-down, it's likely that your immune system is feeling the same effects.

Hopefully, we won't see another pandemic like the COVID-19 pandemic in our lifetimes. But if we do, the preventive measures outlined in the next chapters will help you face not only an unprecedented outbreak but also combat the health obstacles that can arise throughout life.

As I've mentioned throughout this book, you don't need to go cold turkey and implement every recommendation at once. In fact, too much change all at once often leads to more long-term problems down the road. As we discussed in Chapter 4 on change, taking little steps eventually takes us further. And every little step we take toward a healthier lifestyle will help us live our lives to their fullest and longest.

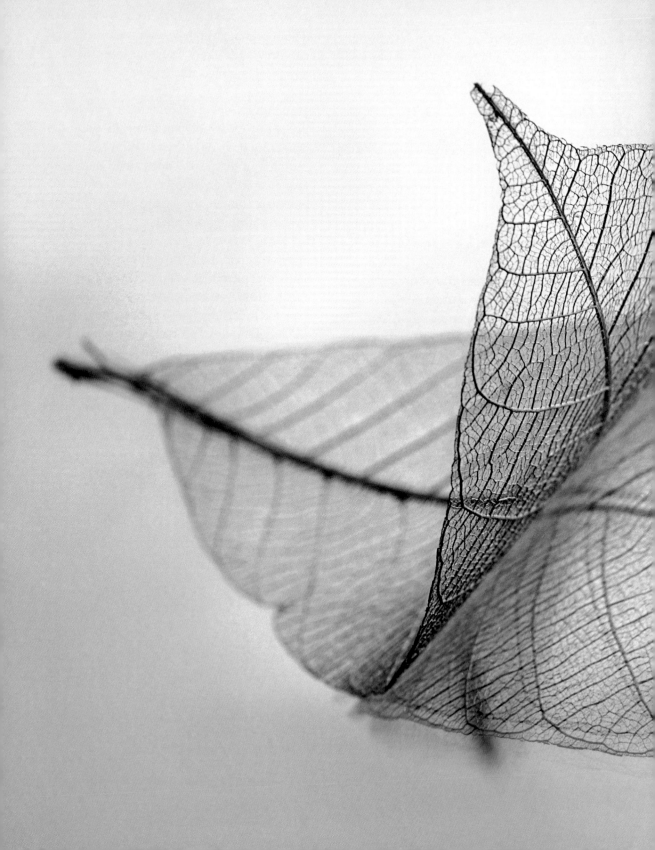

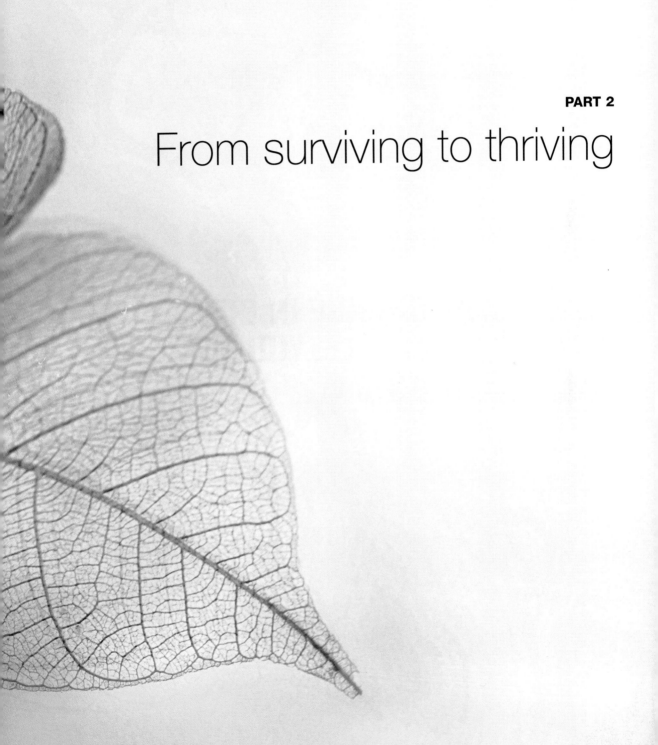

PART 2

From surviving to thriving

NO HEALTHY CHANGE IN DIET IS TOO LITTLE OR TOO LATE. YOU CAN DO IT, ONE BITE AT A TIME.

CHAPTER 8

Step 1: Food that fuels

Diet is the top risk factor for disease and early death worldwide. Heart disease is our No. 1 killer, and what we put in our mouths is the biggest driving force behind it. Diet also has a profound effect on aging and increases the risk of other diseases such as cancer and diabetes.

A 2019 study published in the journal *The Lancet* found that annually about 11 million deaths worldwide are linked to poor diets. And, unlike other risk factors, a bad diet affects people of all ages, male or female, and from all walks of life.

Today we have more food available than ever before. And yet food is proving to be our undoing. Our diets are out of balance. We're not eating enough of the foods that nourish us — fruits, vegetables, legumes, nuts, olive oil and whole grains, for example. And we're consuming too much of the foods that, in excess, put us in danger — a lot of meat, sugar, salt and fat.

One day of eating potato chips and drinking soda may not seem like a big deal. But day after day of consuming manufactured foods that are high in sugar, fat and protein will eventually take its toll. A change in the way we eat is definitely in order, and that's why it's step 1 in reducing our risk of diseases and improving our health spans.

After analyzing dietary patterns across almost 200 countries, *The Lancet* study concluded that if we tweaked our diets, we could potentially prevent 1 in every 5 deaths around the world. Sound ambitious? Maybe. But the good news is that even small changes to how we eat can have a big impact on our overall health.

FOOD AND HEALTH

The relationship between diet and health is powerful. The food you eat can influence your health directly, or it can do so indirectly by way of the numbers on the scale. There's a definite link between excess weight and poor health. Not surprisingly, of the top 10 leading causes of death in the United States, more than half of them are related to being obese or to having an unhealthy diet.

An unhealthy diet lacks key nutrients or it includes generous amounts of animal-based foods or less healthy foods. As an example, consuming red or processed meat — meat that's been salted, smoked or cured — is associated with an increased risk of colorectal cancer, type 2 diabetes, cardiovascular disease and overall mortality.

Some factors that affect your risk of disease are beyond your control, such as age and family history. But what you may not realize is how much you can control your disease risk. While genes may increase your risk of disease 30% to 40%, lifestyle can increase it 300% to 400%. A healthy lifestyle that includes eating well can improve, or even eliminate, significant risk factors for several important chronic conditions. Problems that can develop as a result of diet include:

Coronary artery disease A diet high in saturated and trans fats can increase your blood cholesterol. High blood cholesterol can lead to an accumulation of fatty deposits (plaques) in the arteries that feed your heart (coronary arteries), narrowing the arteries and increasing your risk of a heart attack or stroke.

But limiting saturated and trans fats is only part of the solution. If you want to reduce your risk of coronary artery disease, or even reverse it to some extent, then it's important to also take in more monounsaturated fats, such as those found in olive oil and nuts. If you eat a standard American diet (also called the SAD diet) of saturated animal fat, taking in more monounsaturated fats as part of a Mediterranean diet has been shown to reduce inflammatory signals in your bloodstream and inflammation in your arteries, thus lowering the risk of heart attacks and strokes.

High blood pressure Left untreated, high blood pressure can damage your arteries and increase your risk of strokes and heart disease. Limiting sodium can help prevent or reduce high blood pressure.

Why is this important? Sodium, which is found in salt, absorbs fluid. Have you ever been to a diner and seen a saltshaker on the table with rice in it? The rice is put there to absorb fluid; otherwise the salt would absorb all of the moisture. Clumpy globs of salt in the shaker would make it unusable. When salt circulates in your bloodstream, it absorbs fluid, which in turn raises your blood pressure. The more fluid in a pipe (artery), the higher the pressure.

Cancer Researchers continue to evaluate and clarify the role that diet and nutrition play in the development of cancer. Evidence suggests that about one-third of the cancer deaths in the United States each year may be related to weight or unhealthy habits associated with diet and exercise. Thus, what you choose to eat and drink, along with not smoking and getting regular physical activity, can help reduce your risk of cancer.

Diabetes More than 90% of adults with diabetes have type 2 diabetes, which is primarily due to being overweight and sedentary — conditions that result from a poor diet and lack of physical activity. If you have diabetes, you're also at greater risk of developing cardiovascular disease. Research has shown that weight loss resulting from a combination of a healthy diet and exercise can be almost twice as effective as medication at preventing diabetes in people at risk.

A BETTER PATTERN OF EATING

So what's the answer? To help prevent diseases, it's not necessary to follow a specialized diet, but it's important that you eat a healthy diet. Unfortunately, "healthy diet" has become a hackneyed phrase overused by everyone, including doctors and health experts.

While we know that diet has a powerful effect on health, nutrition can be a complicated topic. It's not always easy to tease out specific associations between health benefits and certain foods. For example, scientists have found that it can be difficult to untangle individual nutrient benefits from a food as a whole.

Vitamin E, for instance, is commonly found in nuts, seeds and green leafy vegetables. It's rich in antioxidants, compounds that help to reduce inflammation in the body. But when vitamin E is extracted from the original foods and made into a supplement form, the health benefits don't seem to carry over as well.

By the same token, the benefits of focusing on a particular food group, such as carbohydrates or protein, are uncertain and unsustainable at best. So there aren't really single magic foods, supplements or food groups that will deliver health to us on a platter.

What research has found, more often than not, is that certain *patterns of eating* tend to be associated with greater health. For example, plant-based diets along with lean proteins seem to have the greatest benefit in terms of preventing common chronic diseases such as heart disease, cancer and dementia. One eating pattern in particular seems to lead to a low rate of diet-related disease.

Eating the Mediterranean way

In the 1960s, researchers started noticing that people living in areas that bordered the Mediterranean Sea, such as Greece and southern Italy, had fewer deaths related to heart disease than people living in the United States or northern Europe. Years of research since have found pretty good evidence that the traditional Mediterranean way of eating has a lot to do with this heart-healthy trend.

Other studies have found that following a Mediterranean-style diet is also associated with a lower risk of developing cancer and dying of cancer, better management and prevention of type 2 diabetes, and a lower risk of dementia.

In addition, the Mediterranean diet improves the number of healthy bacteria in the digestive tract (gut microbiome) and reduces inflammation in the body. Studies also have shown a reduction in:

- Frailty
- Macular degeneration in people 60 years of age and older
- Childhood asthma
- Erectile dysfunction and female sexual dysfunction
- Metabolic syndrome
- Depression
- Fibromyalgia
- Arthritis pain

As a result, the Mediterranean diet is one of several healthy eating plans recommended by the Dietary Guidelines for Americans to promote health and prevent chronic disease.

While no single definition of the diet exists, the typical Mediterranean diet relies heavily on plant foods and follows these kinds of patterns:

- *Daily* consumption of vegetables, fruits, whole grains (not to be confused with multigrain foods)
- *Daily* consumption of healthy fats in the form of nuts, seeds and extra-virgin olive oil

- *Weekly* intake of fish, white meat poultry without the skin, legumes and eggs
- *Limited* amounts of whole-fat dairy products such as a tablespoon of butter a day, or an 8-ounce glass of whole milk
- *Limited* intake of red meat, equivalent to about 3 ounces (or the size of a deck of cards) a day
- *A small amount* of wine, 5 ounces a day for men, 3 ounces for women

While not all of us reside by the Mediterranean Sea — even though we might like to — we can incorporate those aspects of the local diet and way of life into our own lives wherever we are and reap the associated health benefits.

Almost any type of traditional cuisine — such as classic Mexican, Chinese, Indian, Thai or Japanese — can follow a plant-based, Mediterranean pattern of eating.

Anti-inflammatory properties

One of the main health benefits of the Mediterranean diet is its anti-inflammatory properties — the way it helps reduce chronic low-grade inflammation in the body, a condition that underlies so many chronic diseases (see Chapter 2).

Following the Mediterranean diet's focus on fruits, vegetables and whole grains increases the consumption of viscous soluble fiber, which scores high marks for anti-inflammatory properties. Consuming healthy sources of fat, such as olive oil, increases our intake of monounsaturated fats, which also have anti-inflammatory properties. (In contrast, the typical American diet has more saturated fats, which rank high on the pro-inflammatory scale.) Fiber and healthy fats have been found to lower total cholesterol and low-density lipoprotein (LDL or "bad") cholesterol levels.

Fish, another staple of the Mediterranean diet, are rich in omega-3 fatty acids, a type of polyunsaturated fat thought to curb inflammation in the body and reduce triglycerides, blood clotting, and the risk of strokes and heart failure.

Researchers studying the Mediterranean diet and its effects on brain health found an association between eating more fish and a reduced risk of impaired memory and thinking skills (cognitive impairment) as well as a slower rate of cognitive decline.

Such anti-inflammatory properties appear to directly correlate with why a Mediterranean-style diet can decrease the risk of

THE BENEFITS OF FIBER FOR DIABETES

Oftentimes my patients tell me that they can't eat fruits due to the sugar they contain and the adverse effects that will have on their diabetes. Nothing could be further from the truth.

If you're living with diabetes, it's the total amount of carbohydrates, and especially total calories, in your diet that affects diabetes the most. For this reason, you're most likely to benefit from a plant-based diet that's slightly higher in fruits, vegetables and legumes, lower in simple carbohydrates, and higher in healthy fats from olive oil, provided that you take steps to control your daily calorie intake.

The fiber contained in fruits is noncaloric, which means you don't gain weight from it. If you eat an average-size piece of fruit, say a banana or an apple, it contains about 60 calories. But if you eat the equivalent portion of protein, like a chicken breast, you get double the calories, about 120. The same volume of fat is double that of protein, at about 240 calories.

The pulp and fiber in fruits and vegetables provide a lot of filling power, helping you feel full without getting as many calories and reducing inflammation in your body.

EAT MORE THIS, LESS THAT
THE MEDITERRANEAN WAY

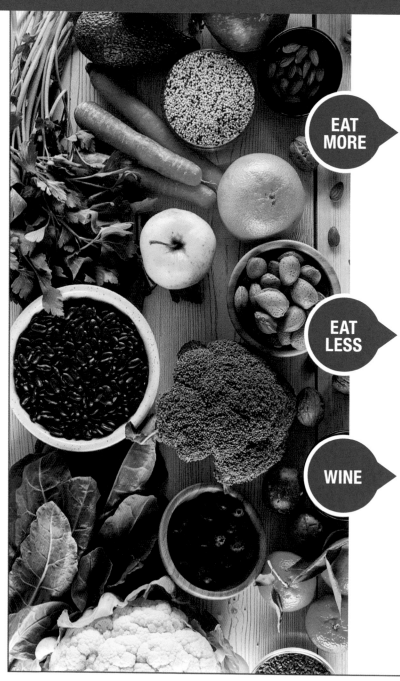

EAT MORE

- Fruits
- Vegetables
- Nuts
- Legumes
- Extra-virgin olive oil
- Minimally processed foods
- Fish and seafood
- Lean poultry

EAT LESS

- Butter
- Full-fat dairy
- Red meat
- Ultraprocessed foods
- Sugary beverages

WINE

Limit to one glass a day
(5 oz. for men;
3 oz. for women)

INSTEAD OF	TRY
Butter or margarine	Olive oil for cooking or dipping whole-wheat bread in
Red meat	A meatless meal, such as one based on legumes (think peas) or beans; vegetable-based recipes Grilled or baked lean, skinless chicken breast; grilled or baked fish or shellfish (tuna, salmon, trout, mackerel and herring are good choices)
Full-fat dairy	Low-fat or nonfat dairy, such as low-fat or nonfat milk, low-fat cheeses, and low-fat or nonfat Greek or regular yogurt; milk alternatives, such as almond or oat milk
Salt	Herbs and spices first, which can eliminate or lessen your need to add salt
Peanuts	Almonds, walnuts, hazelnuts
White bread or pasta, processed cereals	Whole-grain breads, pasta and cereal Alternative grains, such as bulgur and faro
Cream-based sauces	Olive oil-based sauces, tomato-based sauces
Soda, diet soda, juice	Water, carbonated or sparkling mineral water, seltzer, unsweetened tea
Prepackaged, store-bought desserts, cookies, cakes, etc.	Homemade sweet treats (remember, don't deprive yourself; everything in moderation)

death from heart disease, strokes and cancer, and lower your chances of developing diabetes, Alzheimer's, arthritis, Parkinson's disease, macular degeneration, erectile dysfunction and female sexual dysfunction.

More than just a diet

The Mediterranean way of eating isn't focused solely on what you eat. Some experts have proposed that the Mediterranean way of living as a whole offers health benefits.

A traditional Mediterranean lifestyle, not unlike many other traditional cultures of the world, also includes:
• Making an occasion of the meal and its preparation
• Sharing food with family and friends
• Socializing
• Enjoying meals at a leisurely pace
• Frugality
• Moderation in food consumption
• A preference for seasonal, fresh and minimally processed foods
• An emphasis on local products
• Plenty of physical activity
• Adequate sleep

This style of life can be adopted in any culture. One of the key components is to focus on eating as a primary event, rather than an afterthought (think grabbing a burger on the way to the kids' soccer game). Making an event of the meal allows you to eat at a slower pace, which promotes better portion control. There's usually about a 10-minute lag between when your stomach gets full and when your brain realizes it. Therefore, the slower you eat, the less you overeat.

Switching to a Mediterranean-style eating pattern can also benefit our environment. Focusing more on fruits and vegetables and less on animal and dairy products can help reduce a number of risks to the planet, such as greenhouse gas emissions, land use, and energy and water consumption.

Eating a Mediterranean-style diet will shrink your environmental footprint significantly compared to eating a meat-oriented diet. For example, one study showed that moving toward a plant-based diet would decrease agricultural land use by 58%, water consumption by 33%, energy consumption by 52% and greenhouse gas emissions by 72%.

OUR DIETS: WHAT WENT WRONG

In America, abundance, productivity and efficiency have had a large impact on the average person's diet. Even as national experts obsess over weight and nutrition, our eating patterns have primarily evolved around convenience and a taste for sugar, salt and fat.

A lot of people grew up with the "food pyramid," the graphic that arranges all nutritional food groups — vegetables, fruits, grains, proteins, dairy and oils — in order of what you should be eating the most of, all in a tidy triangular shape. The visual here is a bit problematic, as it's natural to think that those foods at the very top of the pyramid are the most important.

In the case of the food pyramid, the opposite is true. The foods at the top of the triangle, occupying a very small space, are those we should be consuming less of, while the foods we need more of provide the larger foundation for the bottom of the pyramid. Unfortunately, it's those foods toward the top of the pyramid that represent what most of us want and, in fact, do eat.

Today, *half of our calories come from sugar, meat and vegetable oil.* Looking at dietary trends since 1961, the percentages of our daily calories that come from sweeteners, meat and oils have increased 17%, 27% and 150%, respectively. Without a doubt the biggest source of these numbers is ultra-processed foods.

Unhealthy convenience

Most food we eat today undergoes some sort of processing. It's not all bad. But it's important to understand the different types of processed foods. Some processing is necessary to make certain foods edible. But extensive processing can be detrimental.

Food items today can generally be placed into one of these four categories, based on the NOVA classification system created by a group of medical and nutrition scientists:

Group 1: Unprocessed (natural) and minimally processed foods Unprocessed foods include such things as the edible parts of plants (seeds, fruits, leaves, stems, roots) and of animals (meat, eggs, milk), and also mushrooms, seafood and water. See the chart below for some examples of foods that have received little to no processing.

EXAMPLES OF UNPROCESSED OR MINIMALLY PROCESSED FOODS

- Fruits and vegetables (fresh, frozen or dried)
- Grains
- Beans and other legumes
- Root vegetables (potatoes, yams)
- Fresh and dried mushrooms
- Meat, poultry, fish and seafood (fresh or frozen)
- Eggs, milk (pasteurized or powdered)

- Fruit or vegetable juices without added sugar, sweeteners or flavors
- Pasta, couscous, polenta
- Grits, cornmeal, flour or oats
- Nuts and other oil seeds
- Herbs
- Plain yogurt with no additives
- Tea, coffee, drinking water

Minimally processed foods are those that have been cooked or slightly altered in some way. By USDA standards, if you heat, freeze, peel, or dice vegetables and fruits, that's considered minimal processing. Other examples of minimally processed foods include unsalted roasted nuts, parboiled white rice, and canned or dried fruits and vegetables. There's no added salt, sugar, oils or fats.

This group also includes foods created from two or more items in this group, such as dried mixed fruits; granola without added sugar, honey, or oil; and foods fortified with vitamins and minerals to replace nutrients lost during processing. These foods are OK to eat.

EXAMPLES OF PROCESSED FOODS

- Canned vegetables, fruits, beans and other legumes
- Salted or sugared nuts and seeds
- Salted, cured or smoked meats
- Canned fish
- Cheese
- Unpackaged breads
- Beer
- Cider
- Wine

Group 2: *Processed culinary ingredients*
These products are extracted from nature and typically used as seasonings. Examples are sea salt, molasses, sugar, honey, maple syrup, butter, cornstarch and pressed oils from olive, sunflower and other seeds.

Some items are combined, such as salted butter, and some have added vitamins or minerals (iodized salt, all-purpose flour) or preservatives (vegetable oils with added antioxidants, salt with anti-humectants, vinegar with microorganism preventives).

Group 3: *Processed foods* These are relatively simple products made by adding sugar, oil, salt or other foods from Group 2 to Group 1 foods. The main purpose is to increase the durability of Group 1 foods, or to modify or enhance their sensory qualities.

Most Group 3 foods have two or three ingredients. When we cook a homemade meal, we are processing foods.

Processed foods also include those that have undergone various preservation methods, such as canning, and in the case of breads and cheese, fermentation. Alcoholic drinks produced by fermentation of Group 1 foods, such as beer, cider and wine, may be classified here in Group 3.

Group 4: *Ultraprocessed foods* These foods undergo a higher level of processing. They're manufactured for convenience and taste. They tend to have at least five ingredients added — usually in high amounts and in the form of sugar, oils, fats, salts and preservatives. Ultraprocessed foods contain little to no natural, unprocessed foods.

Ultraprocessed foods may include substances directly extracted from foods, such as lactose, whey and gluten, and some derived from further processing of food constituents, such as hydrogenated oils, maltodextrin and high-fructose corn syrup. Additives found in this group include dyes and coloring, flavors, nonsugar sweeteners, and various processing agents.

Several industrial processes not found in normal home cooking — and not often heard of — are used in the manufacture of ultraprocessed products, such as extrusion and molding, and pre-processing for frying.

Ultraprocessed foods are ready to consume and hyperappealing to our taste buds. These foods feature sophisticated and attractive packaging, are highly marketed, carry high profitability, and are owned by transnational corporations. A few examples are soft drinks, frozen pizzas, chicken nuggets, instant soups, potato chips, cheese puffs, ready mixes and prepackaged snacks. In fact, ultraprocessed foods account for 58% of the calories we consume.

Ultraprocessed foods in general are very pro-inflammatory foods. Putting ultraprocessed foods in your body can damage it, similar to putting diesel fuel into a car that runs on gasoline, which could seriously damage the engine. Research has shown that these foods should be minimized to no more than three servings a week.

We frequently put foods in our stomach that we were never programmed to eat. I remember asking a farmer who ate a lot of ultraprocessed foods, "Would you put a tank of gasoline into your diesel tractor?" He laughed out loud and said "Gosh no doc, that would ruin my tractor!" So I asked him why he continues to put food into his

EXAMPLES OF ULTRAPROCESSED FOODS

- Frozen pizzas and snacks
- Soft drinks
- Hot dogs
- Prepackaged cookies and chips
- Ice cream
- Ready mixes for cakes and baked goods
- Instant noodles
- Cold cuts
- Margarine
- Microwave buttered popcorn
- Fruit snacks
- Candy
- French fries

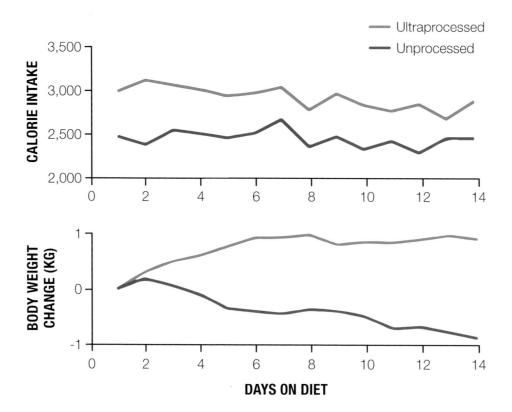

DO ULTRAPROCESSED FOODS LEAD TO WEIGHT GAIN?

In the study illustrated above, 20 people were provided with ultraprocessed and unprocessed diets for 14 days each, in random order. Meals offered from the two diets were matched in terms of calories, sugar, fat, sodium, fiber and other nutrients. Participants were allowed to eat as much as they wanted. When eating the ultraprocessed diet, participants tended to eat more and, as a result, gained more weight than when eating the unprocessed diet. Why did this occur? There are likely multiple reasons but one is that processed foods contain a lot of chemicals called obesogens (see page 107). These compounds may interfere with your metabolism and your body's response to food, leading to weight gain.

Source: *Cell Metabolism.* 2019;30:67.

stomach that his body wasn't designed for. At that his eyes got big and a lightbulb turned on in his mind.

What we eat

Unfortunately, a good chunk of our diets falls into the last category: ultraprocessed foods. When we eat a lot of these foods, it doesn't leave as much room in our diets for the healthy stuff.

Approximately 80% of food that Americans eat is produced in the U.S., and there are seven major subsidized food commodities: corn, soybeans, wheat, rice, sorghum, dairy and livestock. Investigators have found that 56% of calories eaten in America come from these subsidized foods.

These commodities give us some delicious and healthy foods. However, many foods derived from these products are ultraprocessed. In addition, evidence shows that those who eat subsidized foods the most, compared to those who eat only small amounts of these foods, are four times more likely to be obese, five times more likely to have abdominal obesity, twice as likely to have high cholesterol and three times as likely to have elevated blood sugar.

Additionally, we are eating 460 more calories a day now than we did in 1970. Most of the increase is from more flour, more cheese and more fats. Finally, as the figure nearby shows, eating ultraprocessed foods can lead to weight gain in just two weeks.

Research into the effects of ultraprocessed foods on weight and metabolism is ongoing. One aspect that investigators are looking into relates to how chemicals, some of which are found in ultraprocessed foods, may disrupt our bodies' natural metabolic processes.

Chemicals that interfere with the body's hormonal activities are referred to as endocrine-disrupting compounds (EDCs). A subset of these compounds, called obesogens, has been implicated in conditions such as obesity and metabolic syndrome in animal studies as well as in some human studies.

EDCs and obesogens have been found in plastics, pesticides, cleaning products, flame retardants used in furniture and building materials, and personal care products. But they've also been found in artificial sweeteners, phytoestrogens, preservatives and added sugars such as high-fructose corn syrup. It's also been shown that some of the wrappers used for fast-food items contain some of these obesogens. In other countries, such as in Europe, many of these products are limited by law. Unfortunately, the U.S. hasn't followed suit.

Some of the ways obesogens may promote weight gain include changing the way fat cells are programmed to develop, increasing the amount of energy stored in fat tissue, disrupting the body's regulation of when we feel hungry or full, and reducing the rate at which our bodies burn calories. It's possible that these obesogens lead us to eat more calories and metabolize calories more slowly.

CAN FOODS BE ADDICTIVE?

If you've ever struggled to eat just one or two cookies, or one slice of pizza, you know that it can be difficult to not go overboard. You think, "These are so addictive! I must stop!" even while you reach for more. When I was growing up, there was an ad on TV for a very popular processed food proclaiming "Bet you can't eat just one." And they were right, I couldn't. Research on food addiction is ongoing, but what we've learned so far is that the symptoms that surround food cravings do indeed seem to mirror those related to drugs and similar substances.

Hallmarks of food addiction include:
- No control over consumption
- Continued eating patterns despite a negative impact
- Lack of ability to control eating despite wanting to do so
- Hiding it from your spouse
- Planning your day, or going out of your way, to consume a certain food

High levels of ingredients such as refined carbohydrates are most likely to elicit these reactions. Studies involving rats given intermittent access to sugar showed several signs of addiction, such as bingeing and tolerance for greater amounts. When the sugar was removed, the rats experienced withdrawal symptoms, including anxiety, teeth chattering and aggression.

In humans, research seems to point to foods with high levels of sugar and fat as being the most addictive. Brain imaging studies show that such foods light up brain areas associated with a feeling of reward, similar to what happens with drugs.

Food in its natural state rarely seems to create this effect. People don't tend to binge on grapes, carrots or baked potatoes. But greasy, salt-laden fries? That can prove irresistible. As a general rule, the more processed a food item is, the higher its potential for being addictive. And foods that are ultraprocessed tend to be the biggest culprits.

Highly processed foods have artificially increased levels of refined carbohydrates (sugar, white flour) and fat. These may trigger addiction-like responses because they produce unnaturally high levels of reward in the brain. Lots of refined carbs can also increase the rate at which the addictive food components are absorbed into the bloodstream, creating a blood sugar spike. Research has shown a link between blood sugar levels and activation of the parts of the brain involved with addiction.

A food's effects on your blood sugar is often called its glycemic load. Foods with a low glycemic load, such as broccoli or oatmeal, are slowly absorbed. Foods with a high glycemic load, such as cake and ice cream, enter the bloodstream rapidly. Highly processed foods have a high glycemic load because they're the perfect storm of high levels of refined carbohydrates and fat, and little to no fiber, protein or water, which increases the rate of carb absorption.

Not everyone who likes pizza or chips will necessarily eat them uncontrollably. And just because you find yourself craving junk food or even losing control over your consumption of it may not mean you're addicted to it. The Yale Food Addiction Scale — a way to assess addiction-like eating behaviors — found that food addiction often occurs in the context of other issues, such as depression, anxiety, post-traumatic stress disorder (PTSD) and attention-deficit/hyperactivity disorder (ADHD).

A 2015 study published in *PLoS One* ranked foods on their potential to be addictive, with a score of 1 being not at all addictive, and 7 being extremely addictive. As expected, ultraprocessed foods ranked high on the scale. Is it any surprise addictive foods are common in the American diet?

LEAST ADDICTIVE FOODS

- Cucumbers
- Carrots
- Beans
- Apples
- Brown rice
- Broccoli
- Bananas
- Salmon

MOST ADDICTIVE FOODS

- Pizza
- Chocolate
- Chips
- Cookies
- Ice cream
- French fries
- Cheeseburgers
- Nondiet soda
- Cake
- Cheese

What we don't eat

The 2019 study published in *The Lancet* found that more than half of deaths and disability cases related to diet were linked back to a high intake of sodium and a low intake of fruits and whole grains. So what's hurting us is not only what we eat, but what we don't eat.

Take fiber, for example. Hundreds of thousands of years ago, our fiber intake was very high due to the foraging practices of our ancestors. Although current guidelines recommend a daily fiber intake of 14 grams for every 1,000 calories consumed — or about 25 grams per day for women, 38 grams for men — the average fiber consumption of Americans is 17 grams a day. This is problematic because that means we're missing out on all of fiber's benefits. Fiber lowers blood pressure, blood sugar levels and blood cholesterol. And it fills you up on fewer calories.

When consumed in recommended amounts, fiber is linked to prevention of cancer, heart

---

A BETTER CHOICE

Unprocessed or minimally processed foods, in great variety, mainly of plant origin, are the basis for diets that are nutritious, delicious, healthy and anti-inflammatory. Use culinary processed ingredients such as oil and salt in small amounts for seasoning and cooking foods. Eat processed foods such as fruits in syrup, cheeses and breads infrequently.

In general, avoid ultraprocessed foods. Items such as packaged snacks, soft drinks, and instant noodles are convenient and quick. But the way they're produced, distributed and consumed is unhealthy for our bodies and our planet.

Choose natural or minimally processed foods and freshly made dishes along with water and fruits instead of soft drinks, dairy drinks, and cookies or chips. Do your best to prioritize homecooked meals over prepackaged foods and fast-food meals. Choose homemade desserts over commercialized ones.

Finally, minimize cooking oils like canola, safflower, sunflower and corn oil. These oils are ultraprocessed to the point that they have little, if any, of the anti-inflammatory properties that extra-virgin olive oil has.

disease, type 2 diabetes and Crohn's disease. Fiber reduces inflammation in the body, improves the diversity of the gut microbiome (all those healthy, beneficial bacteria living in the digestive tract), helps the body efficiently use calories and nutrients, and boosts the immune system. Not getting enough fiber has been shown to be a leading cause of mortality.

I often ask our students, residents and fellows how much fiber is in red meat. The answer, surprisingly to many of us, is that meat contains no dietary fiber. Fiber only comes from foods that are grown from the ground. Another popular question is how much cholesterol is found in plant foods. Again, the answer may surprise many of us. Nothing that grows from the ground has cholesterol in it.

Where we eat

It's also important to consider where we eat. It's probably not too surprising that we eat out a lot. Whether it's traditional sit-down restaurants or takeout from fast-food joints, we consume one-third of our daily calories eating food prepared at a restaurant. And now, for the first time ever, it's where more than 50% of our food budget goes.

Of course, it's not realistic to cook all of our meals at home. It's nice to go out for dinner or a celebratory meal once in a while. But "regularly" is where we get ourselves into trouble. What are we eating when we eat restaurant-prepared foods? Most likely something unhealthy, according to a recent Tufts University study. At full-service restaurants, about 50% of the meals we consume are of poor nutritional quality. At fast-food restaurants, the numbers are even bleaker (though perhaps not so surprising): 70% of the meals we eat are of poor dietary quality. And how many of these meals eaten out, whether at a fast-food restaurant or a full-service restaurant, would be deemed "healthy" by the USDA? Only 1 out of every 2,000 meals!

Ideally, home is where we would prepare and eat most of our meals. Part of the Mediterranean diet's approach is sitting down and eating with loved ones. It not only feels good to do it, but there are health implications as well, particularly for young people. Research suggests that eating at least three shared family meals per week reduces the odds of being overweight and increases the odds of eating healthy foods for children. Those who eat five or more meals together each week tend to have lower odds of developing eating disorders.

HOW CAN WE CHANGE?

Is it possible to switch from a diet that's built on habit and convenience to one that's more in line with our health goals? Yes, but change doesn't always come easy. It can be difficult to propel ourselves in a new direction.

The hurdles to healthy eating can seem insurmountable at times. Studies show that our taste preferences are formed as early as in the womb, when what our mothers ingested was shared with us via their amniotic fluid. Eating habits are formed early in life, and childhood is typically a landscape dotted with fast foods and sweets.

Grocery stores, where we purchase our food, strive to meet our desires for ease and convenience. Aisles are filled with conveniently packaged, ready-to-eat foods that are easy on our time but not necessarily our bodies. Restaurants offer appetizing dishes that require little of our effort but often come at the expense of a healthy heart and clear blood vessels.

And sometimes, medical experts aren't fully prepared to offer us clear advice. Consider this: Of more than 600 practicing cardiologists surveyed in 2017, 90% report minimal to no nutrition education during their training. The average physician spends 40,000 hours training but only a few spent on learning about diet, now the No. 1 risk factor for early death and disease in our world. In addition, few of our health care dollars are spent on promoting healthy behaviors.

Despite all of these obstacles, you can take charge of your diet. Here's what's important to remember: No healthy change in diet is too little and no healthy change in diet is too late. You can do it, one bite at a time.

Go small, go slow

As humans, we generally resist big, dramatic changes in our daily lives. Think about your breakfast, for instance. On most mornings, it's probably very similar from one day to the next. Maybe it's a bowl of cereal. It's quick and easy and doesn't take a lot of thought.

One day you decide that you really would like to start eating a healthier breakfast every day. So the next morning you make a pot of oatmeal, slice up strawberries and squeeze some fresh orange juice. It tastes great and you feel good, but — that was a lot of effort! And now you're running late for work. The next morning, you decide it's much quicker and easier to grab your bowl of cereal. Plus, you promise yourself you'll find another time to fix a better breakfast. But that time has yet to come.

This is why change is so hard. Change needs to be slow, so that we can tolerate it and so that it can last. And it needs to be easy so that we can do it without burning out. Pulling out all the stops on breakfast may sound like a great idea, but it's probably not doable every morning.

A smaller and easier change might be to pour a bowl of nonsugary cereal and toss in a handful of blueberries. This doesn't take a whole lot of extra effort and is done in a matter of seconds. Once you discover the ease of adding fruit to your breakfast, you might find yourself making it an integral part of the meal.

Or let's say that you'd like to improve your heart health. Your spouse has suggested meatless Mondays, but a meal without meat really isn't a meal to you. Skipping the meat entirely is likely a no-go. So how do you make it easy on yourself to eat less meat? Try eating just a single bite less at mealtime. Every day for a month, eat one less bite of steak or pork or whatever it is, until you become accustomed to eating less. Then maybe the next month, add a bite of vegetables in between your first and second bite of meat. These kinds of changes are much easier to do and to tolerate. And they're much more likely to last.

Chapter 4 has a lot more information on how to make small, lasting changes in your life that will help you succeed in your quest for better health.

Never too young

Children are not immune to the effects of our current way of eating. According to research, preschoolers get more than 40% of their calories from processed or ultraprocessed foods, while 7- to 8-year-olds get almost 50% of their calories from these foods. That's a lot of crackers, chips, cookies, candy, ice cream, soda, sugary breakfast cereals and sweetened fruit juices.

How does this affect their health? For every 1% increase in calories coming from ultraprocessed foods for 3- to 4-year-olds, total cholesterol and low-density lipoprotein (LDL) cholesterol increases by almost 0.5

HOW IMPORTANT IS MILK?

Growing up, we've been told about how important milk is in our diets, helping to build a lifetime of strong bones. But the odd thing is that humans are the only species to still drink it after infant weaning. And in fact, many people find milk harder to digest (lactose intolerance) as they move through their adult years.

So what's the deal with milk? Well, milk is a good source of protein, calcium and Vitamin D. And if you're raising a picky eater, milk can help your child get those nutrients in one place. However, these same nutrients can be found in other foods — dark leafy greens (kale, collard greens, bok choy), salmon, figs and almonds, for example. Plus, we know that drinking too much milk can contribute excess calories; drinking flavored milk, even if it's low-fat, increases intake of added sugars.

So, the short of it is, limited quantities of milk can be part of a healthy diet — particularly if you struggle to get the nutrients elsewhere — but it's not essential.

milligrams per deciliter (mg/dL) by ages 7 to 8. For example, a 3- to 4-year old who consumes ultraprocessed foods regularly and has a total cholesterol reading of 128 mg/dL may see their cholesterol climb to 163 by the age of 7 or 8, a level that's perilously near the upper range of normal (170 mg/dL).

Our kids are growing up overweight and obese — more than ever in the past. It's no secret that carrying excess weight can lead to problems, even for kids. Extra pounds early in life often put children on the path to health problems that were once considered adult problems — diabetes, high blood pressure, high cholesterol, bone and joint issues, sleep issues, and liver disease.

As a family, you can make lifestyle choices that promote healthier habits for yourself and your children. Here are some guidelines to follow for feeding the entire family:

Provide healthy options Keep in mind that ultimately, you decide what groceries come in the house. While it's probably not realistic to deprive your family of all junk food, look for ways to move closer to a Mediterranean-style diet by adding more nutritious foods — such as fruits, vegetables and fish — into your daily menus.

When our children were growing up, Linda and I found foods that they liked and enjoyed eating. We tried to have these available frequently for meals at home. One of our daughters liked eggplant but because she did, her sister didn't. She liked kale instead. Our son liked broccoli. Amazingly, now as young adults they have the same food preferences.

Share regular meals Whenever possible, sit down for a meal together. Sharing a family meal allows parents to model healthy food choices and appropriate portions. It also allows you to talk about your day, share a laugh and offer support. Eliminate distractions such as television and phones to encourage the social aspects of the meal.

Slow down Try to eat at a leisurely pace and enjoy the visual presentation, aroma, texture and taste of the food. Remember, it takes a few minutes for your stomach to have a chance to tell your brain that it's full. If you eat too fast you tend to overeat calories.

Make room for choices Let everyone choose from the healthy options you've provided. This approach not only encourages your child to enjoy mealtime but also helps your child develop decision-making skills.

Let each person decide how much There's no need to be a part of the "Clean Plate Club." Instead, eat slowly and listen to your belly. Help your child discern and heed his or her own hunger and fullness cues. Follow those cues yourself.

Promote flexible eating Flexible eating means no foods are necessarily "bad" or off-limits. Rather, the focus is on moderation and variety. A flexible diet emphasizes healthy, plant-based meals, but allows room for occasional sweets and treats.

Be a role model Your child looks to you for cues on how to behave, including how to relate to food. If you enjoy eating healthy foods, your child is more likely to do the same. If you say, "Wow, these strawberries are so sweet," or "I love how crunchy these carrot sticks are," your child might take the same approach.

When cooking, add a little bit of healthy to the "unhealthy" part of the meal — veggies to the cheesy pasta, for example. As your child observes how you eat and the way you nurture your body and self-image through wise choices, positive talk and a willingness to be physically active, he or she will follow along to the same mental playlist.

Never too old

If you think that you're too old to start eating differently, you might be shortchanging yourself. Adopting a better diet late in life will not only improve overall health, it may even slow down the aging process.

A study out of Spain examined the diets and health of over 2,000 adults 60 and older from 2008 to 2015. Diets were measured according to how well they stacked up to the Mediterranean diet or healthy eating in general. The health index was focused on signs of aging, such as declining ability to function in daily life (functional disability), the existence of chronic illness, deteriorating self-rated health and declining mental health.

The researchers observed that improvement in diet — such as eating less red or processed meat, drinking fewer sugary beverages, and eating more fish — was associated with a decrease in signs of aging, particularly less functional disability. The decrease was such that for every 12 months a person lived, he or she appeared to age only 9 months. How's that for staying young?

The whole package

Proper nutrition is so much more than what you eat or how much you eat. As we've discussed, it's also about how you eat, who you eat with, when you eat, how you cook what you eat, how fast or slow you eat, where you eat, what you are doing while you eat, and how much attention you pay to your food while you're eating it.

These factors have tremendous influence on our eating habits. Anyone who tells you to just eat more of this food (like fat) and avoid this food (like carbs) is usually trying to sell you something and doesn't really understand the multiple factors involved with eating. It's much, much more than what food you put in your mouth.

It's never too late to make changes in the way you choose to eat. Even simple, small steps — such as replacing one bite of red meat with a bite of black beans, for instance — can have a big impact on your ability to live long and well.

BEING PHYSICALLY ACTIVE AND PHYSICALLY FIT ARE BOTH NECESSARY TO OPTIMIZE YOUR OVERALL HEALTH.

CHAPTER 9

Step 2: Be active and fit

I always ask my patients at Mayo Clinic, "What do you do for physical activity?"

The common answer is, "I don't really exercise but I'm busy all the time. I'm always doing something." I tell them that it's good to be busy and active.

Nonetheless, we're a pretty sedentary lot in the U.S. Between work and leisure, American adults spend about half of their waking time — or close to 8 hours a day — seated, reclined or lying down. Europeans aren't doing much better. On average, they spend about 40% of their leisure time, close to 3 hours a day, watching TV.

Science and the way our bodies work tell us that we need two types of physical activity to optimize our health. First, we need to not be sedentary. Let's say you're moving about every 30 to 60 minutes for two or three minutes. By definition, then, you're active (not sedentary), which is beneficial.

But if you never really get your heart rate up, is that enough to keep you healthy and prevent disease? No, it's not, and that brings us to the second type of activity that benefits our health, which is vigorous physical activity. That means doing an activity to get your heart rate up, to breathe heavily or to perspire (and not just due to being outside on a hot day).

This vigorous activity leads to physical fitness. Being physically fit is different from being casually active. Fitness involves performing structured, repetitive forms of physical activities or exercises that improve your endurance, strength, flexibility and body composition.

And yet, working out in and of itself might not be enough, either. If you get up at 5 a.m., go to the gym for an hour and work out, but then sit all day at your desk job, you're still leading a pretty sedentary life. Sitting for most of your day has negative consequences for your metabolism, blood vessel function and other health measures, independent of time spent at the gym or working out. Regular exercise, while important, doesn't seem to overcome the long-term health effects of too much sitting.

The truth is, you need both types of activity. Being physically active and physically fit are both necessary to maximize your health and longevity.

WHY ACTIVE AND FIT?

When we move about, our muscles squeeze or contract to help us walk, run, jump and move our arms around. When muscles contract, they stimulate an anti-inflammatory response set in motion by the immune system. Inflammation, as you'll recall from Chapter 2, can exist at a low-level chronic state in the body and contribute to many different chronic diseases, such as heart disease, lung disease, diabetes and dementia.

Regular physical activity, including exercise, helps to keep inflammation around the body in check. Exercise inhibits the circulation of pro-inflammatory compounds like interleukins, cytokines and others in the bloodstream. These inflammatory molecules damage the lining of the arteries (endothe-

lium), resulting in plaque formation, stiffening blood vessel walls and blood pressure elevation.

Regular physical activity also keeps your body sensitive to the effects of insulin, the hormone that regulates blood sugar levels. You want your body to be sensitive to insulin so that you don't have high levels of insulin traveling through your bloodstream. High insulin levels can lead to inflammation and damage of the lining of the arteries.

In addition, regular exercise helps prevent excess body fat, which is closely linked to bodywide inflammation. When too much body fat accumulates, it ends up getting stored in inappropriate places, such as in the liver and abdomen. Excess body fat, far from being inactive tissue, wreaks havoc on the body, creating a toxic effect on cells. Excess body fat increases inflammation and interferes with insulin efficiency along with many other processes, causing cell death.

Immediate and long-term benefits

Physical activity and exercise have both immediate and long-term benefits. After only 20 minutes of brisk walking, for example, you begin to experience immediate benefits such as lower blood pressure, greater alertness, improved insulin sensitivity, reduced anxiety and better sleep at night.

After several months of regular exercise, your heart and lungs function better and more efficiently (cardiorespiratory fitness), your muscles get stronger, your mood is consistently better with less depression and anxiety, and you're likely to see a sustained decrease in blood pressure. In addition, your immune system is better equipped to fight off infections and tumors.

So how do we get started?

HOW TO NOT BE SEDENTARY

People today move a lot less than they did at the beginning of the last century. At work, where many of us sit at our desks for hours, we're burning an average of 130 fewer calories a day, which, everything else being equal, is almost a pound a month.

We're less active at home as well, where it's all too tempting to park ourselves in front of the TV for the evening. A growing number of us even work from home. And with conveniences like online shopping, banking and socializing, we hardly need to leave the comfort of our chairs.

All that inactivity adds up.

Moving more at work

You don't need to overhaul your entire workday to move more; you just need to be more proactive. If your job involves a lot of sitting, start small. Look for reasons to break up your day by walking around, going to get a glass of water or just stretching for a few minutes before you sit back down.

I have a wonderful job that pays me to sit all day long. The building I work in also has several flights of stairs. I try to take the stairs several times a day to get myself up and out of my chair. And if I move quickly, I get the added benefit of improving my cardiovascular fitness.

I like to take the stairs to a bathroom on a different floor or walk to ask a colleague a question rather than send an email or text message. Some people set reminders to get up and move — maybe walk down the hall for two minutes every hour.

Changing your office setup can also increase your amount of physical activity. If you trade in your chair for a stability ball, you'll activate your core muscles and use more energy by lightly bouncing. If you have access to a treadmill desk or workstation, try to spend at least part of your day working there.

Can this seemingly small amount of activity actually help you? Yes! Studies show that getting up every 30 minutes and walking for two minutes lowers your triglycerides (a type of blood fat), significantly lowers your blood sugar and makes your body more sensitive to insulin.

Moving more at home

At the end of a long day, most of us look forward to some downtime, whether it's watching TV, surfing the internet or playing computer games. Like anything, though,

HOW DO AMERICANS SPEND THEIR DAILY FREE TIME?

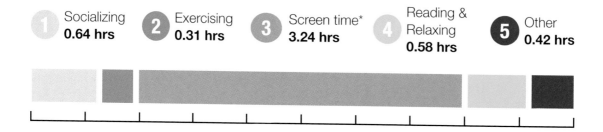

1 Socializing
0.64 hrs

2 Exercising
0.31 hrs

3 Screen time*
3.24 hrs

4 Reading &
Relaxing
0.58 hrs

5 Other
0.42 hrs

To increase fitness, combine exercising and screen time:

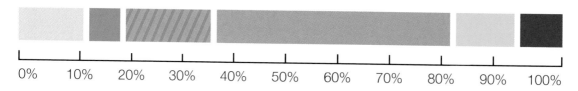

0% 10% 20% 30% 40% 50% 60% 70% 80% 90% 100%

*Screen time includes watching TV and playing on the computer.

Based on U.S. Bureau of Labor Statistics.

moderation is key. Before seeking out that re-cliner, do something to get yourself moving.

Go for a walk around your neighborhood, take 15 minutes to clean up one small section of the garage you've been meaning to get to or sweep two rooms of the house. When doing chores around the house or in the garage, put an extra spring in your step by turning on some music you like.

And when it's time to enjoy that downtime, consider incorporating some physical activity. Stretch, walk on a treadmill or use a stationary bike for an hour while streaming a movie or watching TV. Or get up and move during commercials.

HOW TO GET PHYSICALLY FIT

So you're moving more, but how do you add in physical fitness? Most healthy adults need at least 150 minutes of moderate aerobic activity or 75 minutes of vigorous aerobic activity a week, or a combination of moderate and vigorous activity. You can spread out this exercise during the course of a week. That translates to about 30 minutes a day most days of the week.

It's also important to get some strength training in. It's recommended that you do strength training exercises for all major muscle groups at least twice a week. Activities that promote flexibility and balance, such as yoga and tai chi, also are important, especially as you get older.

This is likely nothing new to most people. Almost everyone knows that they should exercise. Most Americans make a decision every day or two whether to exercise and the decision is usually, "Not today but tomorrow for sure." The issue is finding the time, energy and desire to actually do it. A question I have often contemplated is, what's the most efficient, reliable and convenient way of fitting exercise into my daily routine without taking too much of my time? And how do I make it stick?

My patients are interested in this, too. I'm often asked what is the best form of exercise. Here's what I've found out so far.

What's the best form of exercise?

Clearly, the best exercise is the one that you will do, which usually means the one you enjoy the most, are the best at or have time for. So, if you enjoy jogging on a treadmill, working out on an elliptical, swimming or playing tennis, then do that. There's a great quote, often attributed to Albert Einstein, saying that if we judge a fish by how well it climbs a tree, it will think it's stupid for the rest of its life. In other words, don't keep trying to climb a tree if you were born to swim. Do what you're good at, do what you like to do, do what you have time for — that's the best type of exercise.

Exercise snacks The key to consistent exercising is finding what works in your schedule. As I mentioned earlier, I like to take the stairs in my office building whenever I can just to get away from sitting too long. I also know that if I walk quickly up the stairs, maybe even run up the stairs — five flights or so — I will get in excellent cardiovascular condition. So over the last few years, I've developed the habit of running up the stairs four or five times a day. Going down the stairs doesn't help much and can be very hard on the knees. So I choose just to run up.

I've been doing this for a few years. But just recently I found out that even little bits of stair climbing can benefit my health. A study led by Martin Gibala from McMaster University in Canada, who has pioneered research on how to do the proper interval of exercise with the most benefit to our health, has shown that even brief episodes of climbing stairs are very helpful.

Gibala's lab showed that a quick spring up three flights of stairs three times a day (60 steps at three stairs per second), three days a week for six weeks had a pronounced positive impact on cardiovascular fitness.

To measure fitness before and after the study, the researchers used a test called an oxygen consumption stress test, which we do frequently here at Mayo Clinic to evaluate a person's fitness and risk of having heart disease. In simple terms, the test measures how well your lungs can oxygenate your blood, how well your heart pumps the oxygenated blood around your body, and how well your body tissues can extract the oxygen and use it as energy. It also tells you how much you can improve your stamina.

At the end of the study, participants who climbed the steps increased their peak oxygen intake, compared to those who didn't do stair climbing. In other words, a quick climb up three flights of stairs a few times a day every other day, which doesn't seem like much, really helped their fitness.

The study also showed that going up the stairs faster (three stairs per second) and having less recovery time between each episode (one hour in between rather than two hours, for example) delivered better fitness.

The study called these episodes "stairclimbing snacks," which is a good name since I usually do it when I'm going to our break room to get a piece of fruit or a cup of coffee or a drink. To be honest, it took me months to get to the point where I could run up the stairs without sweating. Or being so short of breath that I had to wait five minutes before talking to a patient so that they wouldn't think I was dying. But it's much easier now than it was in the beginning. And I don't have to make a special trip to the gym to get my exercise in.

It's important to do these fitness bursts regularly. I find that when I'm gone for a long weekend, such as three or four days without going up and down the stairs, it's a little harder for me to do the first day I get back. This is because if we don't use muscles by exercising every few days, the processes don't work as well when we need them to. What do I love most about using the stairs? First, it fits into my daily routine very well and second, my employer pays my salary while I'm doing it! And face it, some days this is all you have time for. But any short, intense burst of exercise can be helpful.

Why are exercise snacks helpful? If you're interested in exercise at all, you've probably heard of interval activity, also referred to as high-intensity interval training (HIIT). It's a way to exercise that's very helpful for our bodies since it replicates what we've been doing on Earth for millennia.

Here's how I describe it to my patients: If you were a caveman hundreds of thousands of years ago, you didn't wake up each day in your cave, turn to your significant other and say, "Honey, I'm going to leave the cave to go jogging for an hour and bring you a latte on the way home."

Of course, there was no latte, but we also didn't go jogging. In order to survive, a lot more was required. And any activity we did was in intervals. What do I mean by that?

Hundreds of thousands of years ago, if we had a language we could communicate in, we would essentially say, "Honey, I'm going to leave the cave, try to find some food, and not be killed." Walking away from the cave, we might see something we wanted to

DOES COUNTING STEPS HELP?

Something I frequently ask patients to do is walk 10,000 steps every day. This has been a popular trend for a while now and it's a good one. You can even download apps on your phone or wear activity monitors that help you measure your steps. But why 10,000 steps?

Because that's right around the number that achieves the greatest reduction in premature deaths before the effects start to level off. A *JAMA* study published in 2020 showed that increasing daily steps reduced the mortality rate from any cause, but more specifically, from heart disease and cancer.

The average American walks just under 5,000 steps a day. Making the change from 4,000 daily steps to 8,000 steps led to the steepest decline in mortality. After about 8,000 steps for women and 12,000 steps for men, the benefits started to plateau. Older adults benefited the most since they're at the highest risk. The study also showed that walking fewer steps, but speeding up every so often, can provide about the same benefit as walking more steps at a steady rate.

STEPS PER DAY AND MORTALITY RATE IN U.S. ADULTS OVER 40

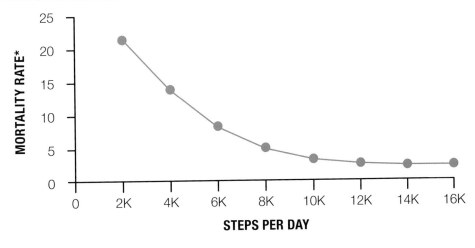

*Per 1,000 adults per year

Based on *JAMA*. 2020;323:1151.

eat, like a rabbit, and chase it. Would we chase it for half an hour? No, of course not. We would chase it for a minute or two and either catch the rabbit or it would get away. Or, some hungry animal might see us and chase us. Would it chase us for 30 minutes? No, of course not. It would either chase us for a minute or two and we would get away — or it would catch us and it would be all over, at least for us.

THE UNFULFILLED PROMISE OF THE GYM

Plenty of people, like me, really aren't that keen on going to a gym and getting on a machine just to sweat. Consider all of the gym and health club memberships that we pay hard-earned money for every month. Most people pay dues like clockwork, but never go. Studies have shown that 63% of gym memberships go completely unused, 82% of gym members go less than once a week, and we use the gym more in the months of January through March than we do in all of the other months combined. Have you ever made a New Year's resolution? The average American breaks it on January 17!

A survey conducted by a charitable organization in the United Kingdom called Better found that while people have good reasons for going to the gym, they also

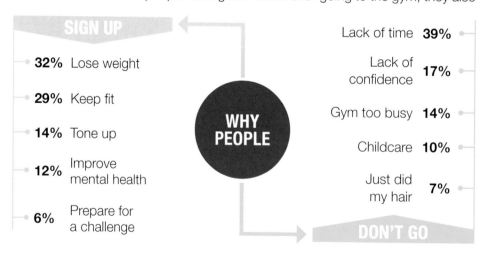

SIGN UP

32% Lose weight

29% Keep fit

14% Tone up

12% Improve mental health

6% Prepare for a challenge

WHY PEOPLE

Lack of time **39%**

Lack of confidence **17%**

Gym too busy **14%**

Childcare **10%**

Just did my hair **7%**

DON'T GO

Based on Top gym excuses. Better. Greenwich Leisure Limited.

What we did long ago was a primitive form of interval training. We would run like crazy to catch our food or run like crazy to avoid being caught for food. We would usually do this for very short periods.

There was no reason for us to run long distances. It didn't help us to survive. All of the activity we did was in short bursts of high-energy activity to maximize survival and minimize energy expenditure.

use a variety of excuses to avoid going to the gym. In fact, money spent on gym memberships is just about the worst investment we make in terms of regular services that we pay for, such as phone service, cable, music or movie services (see chart below). For a gym membership, Americans on average pay 50 times more per hour of use then we do for a popular streaming service. Maybe that says more about our taste for watching movies, but it's also saying a lot about how inactive we are. I remember asking a patient how physically active he was and his answer was, "Doc, I have four gym memberships!" However, he didn't appear to be particularly physically fit and when I pressed him a little harder he admitted that he doesn't go to any of the gyms.

WHAT THE AVERAGE AMERICAN PAYS PER HOUR OF USE FOR:

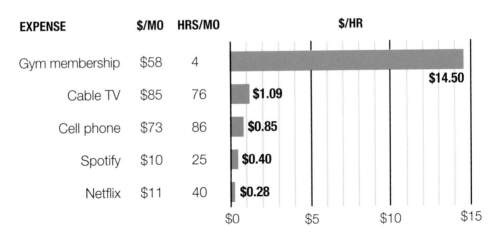

EXPENSE	$/MO	HRS/MO	$/HR
Gym membership	$58	4	$14.50
Cable TV	$85	76	$1.09
Cell phone	$73	86	$0.85
Spotify	$10	25	$0.40
Netflix	$11	40	$0.28

Based on U.S. Bureau of Labor Statistics; Statista.

Survival signals

What's so great about this type of activity? When you challenge your body with short bursts of vigorous activity, your muscles send out several important signals that are key to fitness and to ensuring longevity.

Signal to the heart The first signal is to your heart. The muscles let your heart know that you need to run fast — for all your muscles know, you may be running for your life from a saber-toothed tiger. Regardless, what the muscles do know is that you're asking them to dramatically ramp up activity. The message they send to your heart is that they need more blood to deliver oxygen and carry away waste products.

In return, the heart says, "I can do this, I can increase the blood flow." Our hearts are amazing organs that can increase blood flow sevenfold within seconds by pumping harder and faster. This really is something given that the heart pumps its own blood supply in addition to pumping blood to the rest of the body. Unlike most pumps that plug in to an external power source, the heart generates its own energy supply.

Signal to blood vessels The second very important signal your muscles send out is to your blood vessels. The signal from the muscles is, "The body needs to run fast, possibly for survival. The heart is pumping more blood and you, blood vessels, need to open up wider to allow extra blood through and for waste products to be removed from my muscle cells." Usually, the blood vessels

say, "We can do this." While blood pressure does go up during exercise, this enlargement of the blood vessels actually lowers blood pressure in the long term, which is beneficial for your heart and overall health.

Signal to belly fat The third signal goes from the muscles to our energy storehouse, also known as belly fat. The abdomen is where most of us put those extra calories that we may need to use later but often don't, much to our chagrin. I call this signal "the great American dream" since almost every patient I've ever seen tells me, "Gee, doctor, if I could just lose 5 pounds of belly fat right here, I would really like that."

Why do muscles send this signal to belly fat? Muscle cells don't contain a lot of energy — maybe 20 minutes' worth. The muscles' message is, "I'm working for our survival. If we survive this, the body might want me to run again in an hour and I need to have energy stores ready so I can do that."

To supply the muscles with readily available energy the next time around, the body breaks down belly fat. Each interval primes the body to burn more belly fat so that the muscles have what they need to perform the next time.

Gibala's research has shown that just three minutes of all-out interval exercise three times a week increases your muscles' capacity to extract oxygen and do more work. This improves both cardiorespiratory fitness and cardiometabolic health in overweight adults, and reduces belly fat.

Signal to the clean-up crew The last signal that is sent out with exercise is to the clean-up crew. When we exercise, a certain amount of waste products builds up in our cells. To clear out the buildup, exercise initiates a process called *autophagy* (*auto* meaning self and *phagy* meaning to eat). Autophagy not only cleans up the byproducts of exercise but also does a general sweep of cellular debris, and repairs or recycles damaged cellular components.

Autophagy is a process that's been preserved throughout evolution in all organisms, from yeast cells to humans. Any biologic process that's kept by all organisms is obviously helpful to their survival.

If you could take a pill to clear waste from your cells and help reduce cancers by correcting some of your genetic protein abnormalities, you would say, "Give it to me!" Well, we do have this service available to us and it's called physical activity.

I once told a patient about this clean-up and repair concept. I told him it was "Vitamin E" and he almost jumped out of his chair saying he would buy some and take it every day. I couldn't help but smile when I told him that the *E* actually stood for exercise.

All about survival All of these signals help ensure our survival. To be fast and efficient, the process of responding to these signals requires conditioning. It takes a while for the heart and blood vessels to get in shape to be able to respond appropriately when the need for intense activity arises.

BENEFITS OF INTERVAL TRAINING

1. Heart becomes more efficient and pumps more blood.

2. Blood vessels become wider and more flexible to accommodate increased blood flow.

3. Abdominal fat is reduced by supplying muscle demand for stored energy.

4. Clean-up crew is activated to remove cellular waste and repair damaged proteins.

These exercise intervals must be done regularly, every 48 hours or so, to keep mechanisms in place and working as intended. If a muscle cell isn't being used every 48 hours, it sends out a signal that says, "I'm not being used, don't send me energy — the body doesn't need me." When this happens, muscles get smaller (atrophy). This can happen very quickly, often within days. Unfortunately, it takes months to get back in shape. It's much better to prevent atrophy with regular exercise than to correct it once it does occur.

How do you do intervals properly?

High-intensity interval training is done a bit differently than continuous exercise at a moderate intensity. Continuous exercise is when you warm up, move to a moderate intensity level, and then keep it at that level for 10, 20 or 30 minutes.

There's nothing wrong with the continuous approach. If you're doing it already, that's great and it makes it easier to switch to intervals. But if you're looking for a more time-efficient way to get fit, then interval training might be for you. Interval training is appropriate even for people who are older, inactive or overweight. It's also been shown to be safe and effective for people with heart disease and diabetes. It's all based on your own perception of intensity. You only go as hard as *you* can go, improving as you're able.

You can do interval training with just about any activity. Depending on what you like to do, you can simply increase your speed or other intensity variable such as the incline or tension. For example, you might:

- Go from walking to walking briskly or jogging.
- Alternate between walking and climbing stairs.
- Pedal faster, stand up to pedal or increase the resistance when bicycling.
- Maintain or increase your speed as you run or walk up a hill.
- Alternate between dancing to music that has faster and slower tempos.
- Swim several laps at your regular pace followed by a lap that is faster.

HOW HARD IS HARD?

For an interval session, you should feel that you're working very hard, which is a 16 or 17 on the relative perceived exertion scale. But it's an individual perception. Your perception of intensity probably isn't the same as your friend's. You should be saying to yourself, "Wow, this is really hard and I can't keep this up too much longer."

Borg Rating of Perceived Exertion (RPE) Scale®

6	No exertion at all
7	Extremely light
8	
9	Very light
10	
11	Light
12	
13	Somewhat hard
14	
15	Hard (heavy)
16	
17	Very hard
18	
19	Extremely hard
20	Maximal exertion

© Borg G. Borg Rating of Perceived Exertion Scale. 1998.

EXAMPLE OF A 40-MINUTE EXERCISE SESSION
THAT INCLUDES INTERVAL TRAINING

(1) WALK SLOWLY TO WARM UP
Gradually increase to a moderate pace for five minutes.

(2) WALK BRISKLY
Increase your speed so that you are walking briskly.

(3) INCREASE YOUR SPEED
When you are warmed up, increase your speed or angle so that you are jogging for 30 seconds to two minutes at an RPE of 17 to 18.

(4) SLOW DOWN
Slow down to walking a moderate pace for one to four minutes, or until you get your breath back so you can go just as hard on the next interval.

(5) REPEAT STEPS 2, 3 AND 4

(6) WALK AT A SLOWER PACE
After 35 minutes, walk at a slower pace for five minutes to cool down.

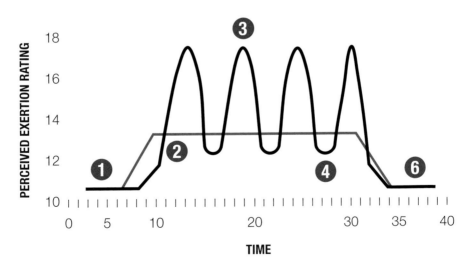

Less is more

The great news is that interval training can significantly decrease the amount of time you need to spend exercising. Dr. Gibala has shown that you can get in the same cardiovascular shape with high-intensity interval training as you would with traditional training, but with less time spent exercising.

Differences can occur in only two weeks. Six sessions of repeated 30-second sprints over two weeks with interval training is equal to 90 to 120 minutes of moderate continuous activity per session. In other words, 11 minutes a day of interval activity can equal 45 minutes a day of continuous moderate-intensity activity in terms of the fitness that you can achieve.

This fact is very helpful for busy people — professionals, parents, college students. Almost anyone can benefit from interval activity, not just in terms of fitness and better health, but also the time spent and the abdominal fat lost.

Benefits of interval training

Interval training has several important advantages, including the following:

Improved cardiovascular fitness Interval training may help you achieve better cardiovascular fitness than continuous exercise. Interval activity increases your ventricular function, which involves the main pumping chambers of your heart. It also improves the function of the tissue that lines your arteries (endothelium).

The endothelium essentially calls the shots in terms of putting out signals to widen or narrow the arteries. A healthy endothelium is essential for those times when we ask our arteries to widen so that we can successfully engage in vigorous activity. (And men, just in case you're wondering, yes, the endothelium plays a big role in controlling blood flow to the penis. A healthy endothelium can help reduce erectile dysfunction symptoms.)

One way to measure progress with interval training is to monitor your heart rate when you exercise. As you get in better shape with interval training, you'll find that your heart rate doesn't go up as much. This is because your heart is getting stronger and more conditioned. It can do the same work at a lower heart rate.

Lowered blood pressure Interval activity leads to lower blood pressure than does continuous activity because of the demand it places on our arteries. This is one of the survival signals that muscles send to the arteries — to widen or dilate during intense activity. Then the arteries stay wide afterward. The bigger the pipe (artery), the lower the pressure (blood pressure).

Increased insulin sensitivity Interval activity leads to increased insulin sensitivity. This is good because it keeps blood sugar under better control and allows lower levels of insulin to circulate in the blood. This in turn reduces the inflammation of the lining of our arteries and hence the development of atherosclerosis, along with subsequent events such as heart attacks or strokes.

Improved physical fitness Interval training allows us to do the same activities we're used to and yet have a lower rating of perceived exertion — the same activities feel easier. It's very satisfying when you see that you can do more than before using the same amount of effort. This is similar to lifting weights and watching your muscles get stronger.

Reduced boredom Interval activity also helps conquer boredom. One reason I don't like to do continuous activity in a gym is that it feels tedious to me. I don't enjoy plodding away on a treadmill. Intervals help break things up, introducing variety into my routine.

Decreased time Many people like doing intervals because the length of time it takes to burn the same amount of calories is much shorter than with moderate-intensity continuous activity. This is a great advantage for people who don't have a lot of time to exercise.

Reduced belly fat Is interval training the magic bullet for weight loss? The truth is, there's nothing really magical about it. It will help you lose abdominal fat if you do it regularly and correctly because your muscles are demanding extra energy from your belly fat cells. This may be the ultimate motivator for people to do intervals and the most enjoyment they get — to see their belt size, pants size or waist size decrease!

Reduced risk of cancer Remember the clean-up crew that helps get rid of waste products and damaged proteins that may carry signals to allow cancers to grow.

If you're sick, recovering from surgery or an illness, undergoing cancer treatment or if you have been very sedentary, be sure to talk to your doctor before starting training.

KEEP AT IT

Being active and fit is a critical component of being healthy. Physical conditioning reduces bodywide inflammation, strengthens the heart, increases lung capacity, builds muscle and widens blood vessels.

In other words, physical conditioning keeps key parts of our bodies in shape, counteracting all of the small daily changes that contribute to aging and disease. Study after study has shown that being active, fit and strong can help us live better and longer. Either we find time now to strengthen and invigorate our bodies on a daily basis or we find time later to deal with chronic illness and disease.

Incorporating short bursts of vigorous physical activity throughout your day can help you get physically fit and keep you from being sedentary. Don't think too hard about it. Just take that first small step and have fun. It can be lifesaving for those of us with a limited amount of time.

SLEEP REJUVENATES US, RESTS US, REPLENISHES OUR ENERGY AND IMMUNE SYSTEMS, AND RESTORES OUR MENTAL SHARPNESS.

CHAPTER 10

Step 3: Prioritize sleep

As busy as we are these days, sleep often seems like an afterthought — something we hope we can get but that isn't particularly high on our list of essentials.

Sleep is a basic necessity, however. It's as fundamental to our health and well-being as fresh air, clean water and nutritious food. There's a reason we spend about a third of our lives sleeping. Sleep allows our bodies to take a break from daytime operations.

Typically during sleep, your body goes into energy conservation mode. Your muscles relax and blood pressure drops about 10% to 15%. Nerve signals that prompt arousal are "dimmed" or "switched off." Brain activity quiets down during most stages of sleep. Oxygen consumption decreases by approximately 10% and your body's core temperature drops.

At the same time, certain restorative activities increase during sleep. For example, brain chemicals perform a rapid clearing of potentially toxic waste products, such as the amyloid beta proteins that are closely linked to Alzheimer's disease. In addition, sleep allows time for cells to repair themselves and for new cells to be built.

Lack of sleep disrupts these key processes, and ongoing sleep deprivation impacts our long-term health. Sleep problems are linked to a number of chronic conditions, including heart disease, depression, high blood pressure, obesity and diabetes — all of the top scourges of health in our world today. Ultimately, this affects our health span and life span.

As humans, we need to do certain things to survive. Every few seconds, we need to breathe; every day or two, we need to eat food for nourishment; every 18 to 24 hours, we need to get some sleep. Most adults need around seven to eight hours of sleep a night.

But many people don't get enough. According to the Centers for Disease Control and Prevention, about a third of adults in the U.S. get less than seven hours of sleep a night.

The time to prioritize sleep isn't tomorrow or this weekend, or even when we go on vacation. Sleep is important now, tonight. After a good night's sleep, we wake up feeling refreshed, alert and ready to tackle the day's tasks. But we're also contributing to a long, healthy life by allowing time for our bodies to restore and rejuvenate themselves on a regular basis.

WHY IS SLEEP IMPORTANT?

Scientists have done a lot of their research on sleep by studying the flip side — what happens when we don't get enough sleep. Sleep deprivation can have a negative effect on practically every system and organ in our bodies.

Brain resources and memory Sleep allows our brains the time to heal and rejuvenate. When we don't get enough sleep, we tend to feel tired and blah. Our brain cells don't communicate as well and our concentration levels decrease, as does our ability to remember. Lack of sleep weakens our reaction times, shortens our attention spans and

leaves us more prone to making mistakes. Even a single night of sleep deprivation can affect our ability to think logically, perform complex tasks and focus on multiple goals simultaneously.

Emotions and decision-making Not getting enough quality sleep also affects our emotions and decision-making skills. Sleep disruption is frequently associated with depression, anxiety and burnout. Lack of sleep can lead to impulsive behavior, poor judgment, irritability and mood swings.

As we go without sleep, our decision-making suffers, including in ways that affect other aspects of our health. For example, evidence shows that for every hour that we're awake during the day, the healthiness of the food we eat decreases by 2%.

Inadequate sleep affects the body in a way that's similar to the effects of drinking alcohol. After 17 to 19 hours without sleep, a person's reaction time, memory, reasoning and hand-eye coordination are equivalent or worse than when having a blood alcohol content (BAC) of 0.05%. For context, consider that most states set their driving under the influence (DUI) limits at a BAC of 0.08% for those over the age of 21. The average legal limit for commercial drivers is a BAC of 0.04%. Driving while sleepy can be just as dangerous as driving under the influence of alcohol.

Immune system When we're tired, even from just one night of poor sleep, brain regulation of the immune system weakens, making us more susceptible to infections. Sleep helps our bodies fight off sickness and feel better. If we aren't sleeping like we should, we are more likely to develop an illness such as a cold or flu. Plus, if we do become ill, we can't fight sickness as effectively and we'll end up in bed for longer than we might like.

Studies show that the relationship between sleep and the immune system is kind of a two-way street. Activation of the immune system by an infection can disturb sleep, but it can also make you sleep longer and deeper, allowing your body to conserve energy for recovery.

Healthy sleep habits are associated with a reduced risk of infection, a better outcome when you do get an infection and a better response to vaccinations. Sleep helps the immune system store information about infectious invaders, including the mild ones introduced by a vaccine. This stored memory equips the immune system to recognize and block the germs the next time they come around. Lack of sleep, on the other hand, can decrease our immune response to vaccinations by 20% to 25%.

The cellular stress caused by a persistent lack of quality sleep can lead to a mild yet chronic activation of the body's inflammatory response. This low-grade inflammation, which we talked about in Chapter 2, is linked to many chronic conditions, including heart disease, obesity, diabetes, dementia and some forms of cancer. Sleep offers our bodies' reparative processes a chance to decrease the daily damage from inflammation. Not getting enough sleep makes for a "double whammy" — not only is our body unable to repair existing inflammatory damage, but more damage piles on.

Heart and blood vessels A lot of evidence supports the importance of adequate rest for the health of your heart and blood vessels. Disrupted sleep leads to changes in blood pressure. High variability in how long you sleep or when you go to sleep is associated with higher blood pressure, abnormal cholesterol levels and insulin resistance.

Not getting enough sleep has also been linked to an increased risk of heart attack. But getting just one additional hour of sleep a night can decrease that risk by 20%, according to some estimates.

The link between lack of sleep and cardiovascular disease is likely caused by the chronic inflammation that poor sleep tends to promote.

Obesity and metabolism Sleep loss can affect your metabolism by impairing your body's sensitivity to insulin and interfering with blood sugar function, which increases your risk of diabetes. Poor or restricted sleep can also impact hormones such as leptin and ghrelin, which affect your appetite. Ghrelin, when increased, makes you hungry, and lack of sleep will increase your ghrelin levels. Disruption of these hormones' normal functions may lead you to eat more than you normally would when you are well rested.

WHAT IS A GOOD NIGHT'S SLEEP?

What does it mean to get a good night's sleep? This is a pretty subjective question, one that's difficult to attach a hard-and-fast answer to. We know that optimal sleep takes into account several factors:

1. **Timing.** This is your sleep schedule relative to the time on the clock. It's also known as process C because of its association with circadian rhythms — your internal body clock that coordinates your sleep and wake times with the 24-hour day-night cycle.
2. **Duration.** This is the number of sleep hours your body requires to be rested or in balance. This is also known as sleep homeostasis or process S.
3. **Quality.** Quality sleep is sound, uninterrupted sleep. Poor sleep is fragmented or disrupted sleep. Sleep can be disrupted by difficulty falling asleep, waking up frequently in the night and having trouble going back to sleep.

How much sleep each of us needs varies from person to person. But in general, seven to eight hours of sleep is the amount most people need to feel rested and is the amount associated with the lowest mortality risk.

If you don't feel refreshed on waking in the morning and you're feeling tired or sleepy during the day, especially when you're not required to physically or mentally exert yourself, then you're probably not getting enough sleep, your sleep is fragmented or your timing is off. A good tip to follow: Try to wake up without an alarm clock. If you need an alarm to wake up, you may not be getting enough sleep.

Good sleepers vs. poor sleepers

Although scientists don't know the exact definition of a good night's sleep, they have observed differences in sleep patterns related to timing, duration and quality that can have an effect on your health.

WHAT ABOUT OCCASIONAL NIGHTS OF BAD SLEEP?

Sleep duration is typically measured using the average number of hours a person sleeps over a certain amount of time. But there are many people who, every so often, don't get enough sleep or sleep poorly. If their average sleep duration is within healthy ranges but they don't compensate for those intermittent nights of poor sleep, they're still building up a sleep deficit, along with the health consequences that accompany loss of sleep.

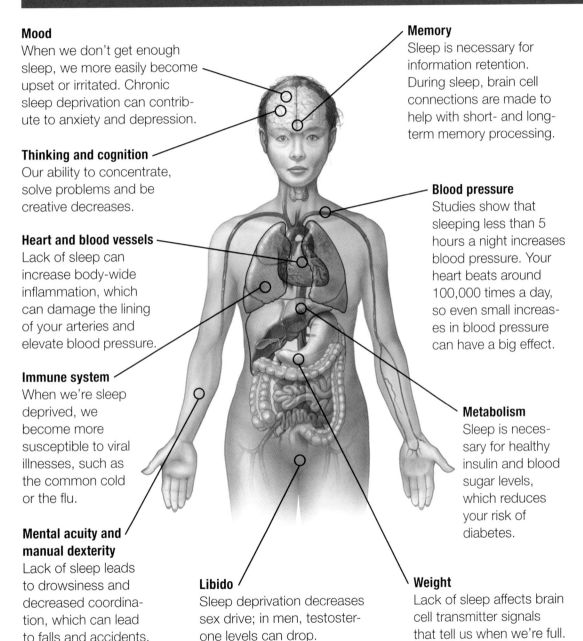

Mood
When we don't get enough sleep, we more easily become upset or irritated. Chronic sleep deprivation can contribute to anxiety and depression.

Thinking and cognition
Our ability to concentrate, solve problems and be creative decreases.

Heart and blood vessels
Lack of sleep can increase body-wide inflammation, which can damage the lining of your arteries and elevate blood pressure.

Immune system
When we're sleep deprived, we become more susceptible to viral illnesses, such as the common cold or the flu.

Mental acuity and manual dexterity
Lack of sleep leads to drowsiness and decreased coordination, which can lead to falls and accidents.

Memory
Sleep is necessary for information retention. During sleep, brain cell connections are made to help with short- and long-term memory processing.

Blood pressure
Studies show that sleeping less than 5 hours a night increases blood pressure. Your heart beats around 100,000 times a day, so even small increases in blood pressure can have a big effect.

Metabolism
Sleep is necessary for healthy insulin and blood sugar levels, which reduces your risk of diabetes.

Libido
Sleep deprivation decreases sex drive; in men, testosterone levels can drop.

Weight
Lack of sleep affects brain cell transmitter signals that tell us when we're full.

A good or regular sleeper is one who goes to bed and wakes up at regular times, needs fewer than 15 minutes to fall asleep, and spends fewer than 15 minutes awake during the night on five or more nights per week. A good sleeper's sleep duration varies by only about 10 minutes every night.

A poor or irregular sleeper's schedule, on the other hand, is all over the place. A poor sleeper goes to bed at differing times and often takes a long time to fall asleep. Wake times also vary and total time asleep can vary by a couple of hours or more.

CAUSES OF POOR SLEEP

We know that not getting enough quality sleep can affect our health in many different and important ways. But what causes poor sleep in the first place?

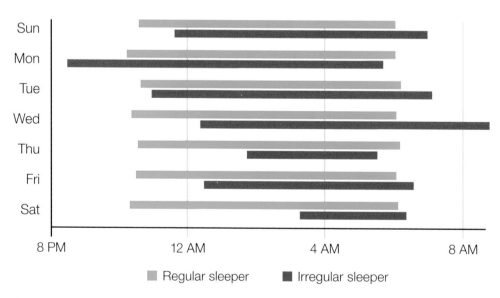

HOW YOUR SLEEP SCHEDULE AFFECTS YOUR HEART

The rhythms of your heart and circulatory system are closely tied to your body's circadian and sleep rhythms. A regular sleeper goes to bed at about the same time

Source: *Journal of the American College of Cardiology*. 2020;75:991.

Circadian disruption

The circadian rhythm is the body's internal clock, which runs on roughly a 24-hour cycle. It's the dominant influence on our sleep-wake cycle and is strongly influenced by the amount of light in the environment.

The lighter and brighter your surroundings, the more awake and alert you are. The darker your environment, the more melatonin — a substance that makes you drowsy — your body produces. Natural circadian rhythms explain why most people are awake when the sun is up and feel sleepy after the sun goes down.

Receiving little daylight or living in a perpetually dim environment can put your circadian rhythms in limbo and interfere with nighttime sleep and daytime functioning. Getting plenty of sunlight during the day

every night and sleeps for about the same number of hours. An irregular sleeper goes to bed at varying times and sleeps for irregular amounts of time.

An irregular sleep schedule can disrupt your cardiovascular rhythms and put you at higher risk of cardiovascular disease (CVD). The higher the variability in how long you sleep (duration) or when you go to sleep (timing), the greater your risk.

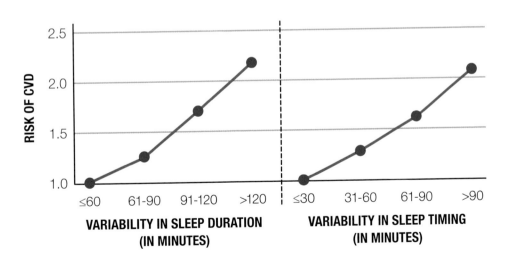

can help synchronize your biological clock with the course of the day and promote better sleep.

On the other hand, lots of light exposure after dark can inhibit the production of melatonin and keep you awake longer than you would be naturally. Light exposure might come from a range of sources, from personal electronic devices to working the night shift. If you can lessen your exposure to light around nightfall, you can allow your mind and body to more naturally prepare for bedtime.

Dawn of the internet

Do we believe we're getting enough sleep? Gallup has annually polled Americans about sleep for decades. Over this period, the perception that we get as much sleep as we need has decreased steadily while the belief that we would feel better with more sleep has increased. This trend started in the early 1990s, right around the time when the internet started to become more widely available to the public.

What does the internet have to do with our sleep? Well, for as far back in time as we can tell, humans have been programmed to go to sleep when it gets dark and wake up when it gets light. This has changed relatively recently due to the incandescent light bulb, but the era of electricity represents a tiny amount of time compared with the number of years humans have been on earth.

This sleep-wake rhythm is driven primarily by blue light from the sun (which also makes the sky look blue). When we look at digital screens, especially our smartphones, we're exposed to an artificial form of blue light. When we look at our screens early in the night, we delay our circadian rhythms so that we stay awake and go to sleep later. However, when we look at our screens late in the night, we actually shift our circadian rhythm so that we wake up earlier. This leads to disruption of our sleep due to the early wakening and subsequent sleepiness the following day. You can buy blue-light filter glasses but these only block a little over half of the blue light, so the phase shift effect persists.

Lack of prioritization

Another issue is how we approach sleep. Is it a priority for us? Lack of sleep is similar to stress in that both are so common that they have become the norm. We tend to view chronic sleep deprivation as a part of modern life. As a result, the importance of sleep has diminished. A poll run by the National Sleep Foundation has shown that sleep is way down on the priority lists of most Americans. It ranks behind fitness and nutrition, work, and hobbies, with only 10% of Americans feeling that sleep is a priority.

Modern living

Many aspects of our current lifestyles contribute to lack of sleep.

Digital entertainment Often, we lose out on getting enough sleep because we work long hours and we're tempted by always available entertainment on our TVs, phones or other electronic devices. So we stay up late watching a favorite show or scrolling through social media, yet still need to get up to get to work or school on time the next day.

Stress and anxiety Going to bed with your mind filled with lists of things you failed to accomplish that day or things you need to do the next day can keep you from falling asleep or wake you up in the middle of the night. If you allow yourself to dwell on things that are weighing on your mind or making you anxious, you don't allow your brain to sufficiently relax to get quality sleep.

Caffeine Caffeine in drinks such as coffee or soda can interfere with sleep as well. Some people are more sensitive to caffeine than others. If you find that drinking caffeine in the afternoon and evening keeps you up at night, you may need to limit it to mornings.

Alcohol Consumption of alcohol before bedtime, particularly in great amounts, may make you fall asleep faster, but it has a tendency to produce more-fragmented sleep. Clear-cut distinctions in drinking habits between poor and good sleepers don't always exist. But if even moderate to minimum use of alcohol seems to disrupt your sleep, it may be worth avoiding it to see if your sleep improves.

Medications Some prescription medications — including steroids, some high blood pressure medications and antidepressants — can interfere with sleep. Many over-the-counter medications, including some pain relievers, decongestants and weight-loss products, contain caffeine and other stimulants.

Late-night dining Eating a heavy meal before bedtime can increase your risk of digestive discomfort, which can keep you awake. If you're often in the habit of eating a large dinner and then having to wait for indigestion to pass before you can fall asleep, try going for lighter dinners that are more conducive to lying down and sleeping. You may have noticed that eating lots of processed carbs will lead to sleepiness. Some people do this to try to help them get to sleep but it's not a viable long-term strategy.

Sleep problems

Some of us have more-specific sleep problems, such as insomnia, obstructive sleep apnea or a snoring partner. It's important to get these sorts of sleep problems evaluated by a doctor so that they can be treated appropriately and you can get the rest you need for your health (and, in many cases, the health of your partner).

Obstructive sleep apnea, for example, is a condition that causes the muscles in your throat to relax repeatedly during sleep. This blocks your air passage and interrupts your breathing. It's characterized by loud snoring, pauses in breathing during sleep, and waking up gasping or choking. It can be treated effectively with therapies such as positive airway pressure (continuous positive airway pressure or CPAP is common) or an oral device to hold your throat open. It also helps to follow the steps outlined in this book — eating well, exercising, not smoking, reducing stress and minimizing alcohol. These steps can all help treat obstructive sleep apnea.

Insomnia is another common sleep problem. Insomnia makes it hard to fall asleep, stay asleep or both. It can cause you to wake up too early or not be able to get back to sleep. Most of the time, simple changes in your daily habits — such as a regular sleep schedule, using your bed only for sleep or sex, keeping your bedroom dark and comfortable, and having a relaxing bedtime routine — can help minimize sleepless nights.

Cognitive behavioral therapy for insomnia is a type of talk therapy that can help you reframe your mindset about sleep and teach you how to develop good sleep habits. In some short-term cases of insomnia, medications can be helpful.

HOW TO GET BETTER SLEEP

Knowing that sleep is key to sustaining our short- and long-term health can help us prioritize a healthy sleep schedule. We can even treat getting enough sleep as being on the same level of importance as taking a medicine for asthma or high cholesterol. Sleep is as vital to health and healing as any

drug, vitamin or herbal supplement, and probably even more so.

Sleep is when the body rejuvenates, repairs and replenishes itself. When we don't allow that to happen properly, our bodies age quicker and we develop noncommunicable chronic diseases earlier in life. Like any medicine, sleep must be taken regularly. To make the most of your nightly "dose" of sleep, consider these important factors.

Getting to bed on time

Even when we understand the importance of sleep, our bedtime schedules can be crowded back by all of the other events that fill our evenings. Our actual bedtime may stem from habits that develop earlier in the day. Relaxing after work, making dinner for the family, fitting in loads of laundry or watching TV are all habits that we can develop in the late afternoon and early evening.

And there's nothing wrong with these habits — they help close out the day and wrap up daily goals. All too often, though, these seemingly important habits encroach on bedtime, narrowing down the time allotted to sleep. If we're not careful, sleep ends up last on our list of priorities.

As with other changes we might want to make, we need to set ourselves up for success. We start small, we do things we enjoy and we make it easy on ourselves. We don't want to ditch healthy meals or time spent together with our loved ones. But we can tweak things here and there — start dinner a little earlier, divvy up tasks or limit our TV viewing to one episode of a series instead of two or three — to achieve a reasonable bedtime.

The benefit of rituals

For most of us, switching from daily activities to nightly slumber isn't an immediate thing. We need rituals in between to help us make that transition. An hour or so before bedtime, we can start to slow down and get ourselves ready for the rest our bodies so richly deserve.

You might already have your own preferred bedtime rituals. Maybe this involves getting kids into bed, prepping coffee for the morning, reading with a cup of tea, brushing teeth or getting into comfortable pajamas. We all vary in our bedtime rituals.

The goal is to signal to our brains that rest is imminent. Because brain activity is so integral to sleep, it's important to get the message through. We need to tell our brains that the day's labor is done and that outlying stressors and anxieties can be set aside until tomorrow. Allowing our brains to relax sends messages to the rest of the body that the restorative functions of sleep can now take place.

WHEN DISRUPTED SLEEP IS THE NORM

If you struggle with falling asleep or staying asleep, you can start to develop negative as-

SLEEP CHECKLIST

- [ ] Cut back on caffeine if needed.

- [ ] Get enough daytime exercise.

- [ ] Avoid heavy meals before bed.

- [ ] Reduce screen time an hour before bed.

- [ ] Relax with a bedtime routine *(for example, gratitude meditation, practicing optimism, journaling or reading)*.

- [ ] Cool bedroom temperature.

- [ ] Keep room dark, comfortable.

- [ ] Take slow, deep breaths.

sociations with sleep. If these associations persist, they can create a harmful cycle that leaves you chronically sleep deprived. Negative associations can develop around your nightly habits before bed, the sleep environment in your bedroom or the process of falling asleep.

Negative conditioning created by the way you prepare for bed or approach bedtime may in fact increase your brain's alertness and make it very difficult to fall asleep.

Say, for example, that you always are late to bed, which increases your worry that you won't get enough sleep before the next day. In your rush to get to sleep, you ignore bedtime rituals and jump straight in between the sheets. Once there, though, your brain is so wound up that you're nowhere near feeling drowsy. You toss and turn, but sleep remains elusive. Once again, you've failed at getting a good night's rest. The next night, your brain remembers the difficulty falling asleep, and the whole process reignites. Remember the habenula, the tiny reward center in your brain that we talked about in Chapter 4? It's keen to remember failure

---

3 WAYS TO RELAX YOUR BRAIN BEFORE BED

Evidence indicates that one of the behaviors most strongly associated with poor sleepers is the habit of ruminating about important matters at bedtime or right after getting into bed. Finding ways to clear your mind at bedtime can produce substantial sleep improvement. Here are three techniques to try:

1. **Gratitude practice.** I like to practice a ritual of being thankful for three things at the end of my day before I go to sleep. This increases optimism and, if practiced regularly, reduces the risk of heart attack after a few years. Focusing on gratitude also relaxes me and helps me forget about the things I didn't get accomplished that day.
2. **Mindfulness meditation.** This stress-reduction technique can be so simple that people often don't realize its effectiveness. The idea is to cultivate an acute awareness of the present moment and to let go of everything else. Focusing your awareness onto the sensations of becoming at rest — the sinking of your body into the bed, the softness of your pillow, the slowing of your breath — and keeping it there helps to dissipate stressful thoughts about other things.
3. **Schedule worry time.** If worries about work, school, family or other concerns keep you awake at night, try to deal with them before bedtime. Set aside a dedicated time when you write down your concerns and then brainstorm possible solutions. That way you have your list ready for the next day, and you can face it with a fresh, rested perspective.

and will remind your body that this sleep business is a not a feel-good situation. And so you'll begin to avoid it more and more.

To undo this cycle, you need to expose your brain to the glow of success. And to do that, you need to break the conditioned responses that happen when you repeatedly try to sleep without success. How do you do this?

Refresh your bedtime rituals They don't have to take up a lot of time, but you do need a few rituals signaling bedtime, such as brushing your teeth or getting into proper pajamas. Relax your mind by reading a book, contemplating a few things you're grateful for or focusing on slowing your breathing. Do your best to go to bed at the same time every night and wake up around the same time every morning.

Reclaim your bedroom Only use your bedroom for sleep or sex. Remove prompts for activities that don't belong in the bedroom, such as watching TV, working on a computer or browsing apps on your phone. It may also help to remove pets from the bedroom. If you can't sleep, get up and go read a boring book or magazine in an upright chair. Do this until you start to feel very sleepy, and then go back to bed. The important thing is that you don't want to associate your bed with not sleeping.

Rinse and repeat You'll likely need to do this routine repeatedly until your brain starts to feel good about bedtime and sleeping. The trick is to make it easy to fall asleep but hard to do other things like worry, watch TV or anything else that will hype your brain.

Sleep's halo effect

Although getting more sleep may seem like the least urgent change you need to make in your life, the truth is that quality sleep creates a halo that touches all other areas of your life. When you're rested, you make better choices about what to eat and how much to eat, you have more energy for physical activity and exercise, you're more patient and attentive to those around you, you're less prone to getting sick, and you're mentally better equipped to handle stressors, large and small. So don't put off sleep any longer — seize the night!

MANY OF US ARE LIVING WITH TOO MUCH STRESS, AND THAT CAN TAKE A SERIOUS TOLL ON OUR PHYSICAL AND EMOTIONAL HEALTH.

CHAPTER 11

Step 4: Get a handle on stress

You're stuck in traffic, worrying that you'll be late for an important meeting at work. With nothing to do but stew in your car, you start ruminating on other worries — a thorny work project, an unexpected medical bill, an upsetting story you saw on the morning news.

We've all experienced stressful moments like this. They're so common that many of us think they're unavoidable. You might not like all the stress in your day, but that's just life, right? Or maybe you think stress is good. I've had patients tell me, "Doc, stress is my middle name" or "Stress is what gets me up in the morning" or even "I don't get stressed — I give stress."

It's true that some amount of stress in our lives is not only normal but helpful. Short-term stress can motivate us to meet a dead-line, confront a family crisis or stop a toddler from running into the street. But many of us are living with too much stress, and that can take a serious toll on our physical and emotional health.

In today's world, there's no shortage of stressors. A recent survey by the American Psychological Association identified some of the most common sources of stress. They range from fears of mass shootings and worries about the economy to concerns about health care, work-related pressures and personal finances.

Most recently, we've all been reminded of the power of historic events to disrupt lives, causing additional stress and anxiety. The rapid spread of the COVID-19 virus across the globe starting in 2019 left many people in an extended state of uncertainty and worry.

Stress can be chronic as well as sudden in the way it affects us.

Regardless of the sources of our stress, most people feel they experience too much of it. This is especially true for younger generations. Those born in 1997 and onward, also known as Generation Z, report the highest levels of stress, followed closely by millennials and Generation Xers.

The good news is that you can learn to tackle stress — even sudden, large amounts of stress — by engaging in small, daily habits that keep stress from becoming overwhelming or taking over. Stress may be a fact of life, but it doesn't have to rule your life. Learning healthy ways to react to and relieve stress can have profound effects on your health, longevity and well-being.

YOUR BODY ON STRESS

Hundreds of thousands of years ago, we humans encountered stressful life-or-death situations on a regular basis. Our bodies were hard-wired to react to predators, aggressors and other immediate threats quickly and effectively. Although these types of threats are much rarer today, our bodies' natural stress response hasn't changed.

When you encounter a perceived threat, such as a large snarling dog, an alarm system known as the hypothalamic–pituitary–adrenal (HPA) axis activates in your body. This system starts with the hypothalamus, a tiny region at your brain's base.

The hypothalamus prompts the pituitary gland just below it in the brain to send a signal to your adrenal glands, located atop your kidneys. The adrenal glands then release a surge of hormones, including adrenaline and cortisol.

Adrenaline increases your heart rate, elevates your blood pressure and boosts energy supplies. Cortisol, the primary stress hormone, increases sugars (glucose) in the bloodstream, enhances your brain's use of glucose and increases the availability of substances that repair tissues.

Cortisol also curbs functions that would be nonessential or detrimental in a fight-or-flight situation. It alters your immune system responses and suppresses your digestive system, reproductive system and growth processes. The stress response also affects the regions of your brain that control mood, motivation and fear.

This complex natural alarm system empowers your mind and body to react quickly to a perceived threat with a fight, flight or freeze reaction. Once the perceived threat has passed, hormone levels return to normal. As adrenaline and cortisol levels drop, your heart rate and blood pressure return to baseline levels, and other bodily systems resume their regular activities.

The dangers of chronic stress

The body's fight-or-flight response to a short-term threat is called acute stress. Acute stress serves an important role in keeping you safe and overcoming immediate challenges. But what if a source of stress isn't a short-term threat you can resolve with quick action? What if you're dealing with a complicated problem at work or an ongoing difficulty at home? These daily stressors may be turning on the stress response — and keeping it on.

When stressors are always present in our lives and we constantly feel under attack, we're likely to experience chronic stress. The effects of chronic stress are often more subtle than acute stress, but they may be longer lasting and more problematic.

Chronic stress leads to the long-term activation of the stress-response system. The result is overexposure to cortisol and other stress hormones that can disrupt almost all of the body's processes. This can put you at increased risk of health problems and unhealthy habits that may impact the quality and length of your life, including:

Heart disease When you're stressed, your blood pressure and heart rate go up and your heart contracts more forcefully. Stress also increases inflammation of the arteries that supply blood to your heart.

In Chapter 2 we talked about how the lining of your arteries (endothelium) is like wallpaper, but that it doesn't just sit there — it's biologically very active. The endothelium helps control the arteries' ability to widen when more blood is needed to supply the heart in times of stress.

The endothelium is also where heart attacks begin. Anything that damages the endothelium — such as high blood pressure, smoking, excess cholesterol or stress — leads to erosion or a tear in the lining with subsequent blood clotting. This can dramatically restrict the flow of oxygen-rich blood to the heart muscle.

Impaired brain function Stress can impact your ability to think clearly, learn new information and store memories. Some research suggests that stress may increase the risk of certain forms of dementia, including Alzheimer's disease.

Weakened immune system The hormones your body releases under stress may interfere with or suppress your immune system. Studies have shown that chronic stress causes your body to have a harder time fighting off infection, such as the common cold or flu, and even limits the effectiveness of flu and shingles vaccines.

Anxiety and depression Living with constant stress can be exhausting and dispiriting, leading to anxiety and depression. Some research suggests that chronically elevated levels of stress hormones may also contribute to the development of mood disorders.

Digestive problems Stress can cause nausea, diarrhea and gas, along with pain and bloating in the stomach and bowels. Over time, chronic stress may lead to chronic bowel disorders, such as irritable bowel syndrome (IBS) or inflammatory bowel disease (IBD).

Unhealthy behaviors When you're under constant stress, it's easy to let good habits fall by the wayside. You might skimp on sleep, eat too much or too little, and exercise less often. Studies have shown that when we can't adequately manage our stress, many of us tend to eat more junk food. Other responses to stress may include using tobacco products, misusing drugs or alcohol, and withdrawing socially from friends. These behaviors can take a serious toll on your health and well-being.

Diabetes Chronically high levels of stress hormones can interfere with your body's ability to use insulin properly, which may lead to greater insulin resistance. This can increase your risk of developing type 2 diabetes or make already existing diabetes harder to manage. Plus, the excess insulin in

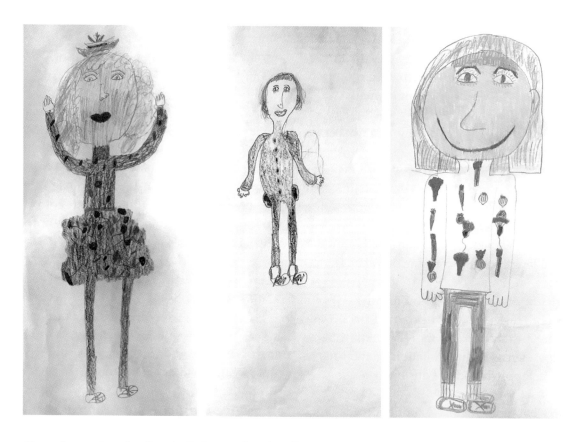

Above is a series of self-portraits by my daughter Emily that vividly portray the effects of stress and how we eventually adapt. Note the changes from one drawing to another, starting from the left, drawn before my second cancer diagnosis, right after the diagnosis, and two months after the diagnosis. Note the change in color, size and confidence in the middle one.

your bloodstream leads to damage of the endothelium with subsequent increased risk of heart attack and stroke. The problem may be compounded if stress is negatively affecting your eating and exercise habits.

Weight gain Overeating and underexercising can cause you to gain weight. Elevated cortisol levels activates your body to store more fat, increasing your risk of obesity. When the body is stressed, the response is to store away calories as fat in preparation for upcoming fight-or-flight scenarios, which in the past were typically physical events requiring lots of extra energy. Hundreds of thousands of years ago, this mechanism helped us survive. But now it actually works against us by storing away extra calories that we don't use.

MANAGING STRESS

Since we're all different, stress is different for each of us. What causes stress in one person might not cause stress in another.

And there are different kinds of stress. Some stress is actually good stress, such as when competing in a sport with friends. Win or lose, you tried your best and had fun, coming away feeling energized. Some stress is manageable, like the stress of driving and getting slowed by a stoplight that lasts longer than we'd like. In the big picture of life, it's not important. But some stress can be toxic. This is the kind of stress where you have little to no control, such as in the death of a loved one or a large personal financial

crisis you can't change. With toxic stress, it's critical to have help and support from family or professionals. It also helps if you've learned how to deal with stress in positive ways during your early years of life.

But it's never too late to learn. There is great benefit, and subsequent satisfaction, in finding ways to deal with stress.

That's where the next step of stress management comes in — learning more-effective ways to respond to stress. There are three basic approaches we can take when faced with one of our stressors: change our environment, change how we react or change both.

In most cases, it's not practical to make drastic changes to our environment. We can't simply switch jobs, swap families or go on a big vacation every time stress rears its head. But we can react to stress more effectively by incorporating small habits into our daily lives. Adopting even one new healthy habit and practicing it each day can help to fight the harmful effects of stress.

When I had my second cancer, I was married with three children and a full-time job as a cardiologist at Mayo Clinic. Aside from the cancer, it really was a dream come true for me. When I started chemotherapy, I wanted to keep working but found it difficult because of the chemotherapy's side effects. Although Mayo Clinic was wonderful in helping me deal with my work situation, the guilt I felt from my inability to work took a tremendous mental toll on me and actually diverted my energy away from focusing on healing my cancer.

I visited with a chaplain, a Roman Catholic priest, who suggested that I have what he called a "board of directors meeting" that night in my mind, with me as the chairman. He suggested I assemble the board around this imaginary table and address each member individually. I should explain why I could not work full time but instead why I needed to focus on curing my cancer.

When I asked him who I should have around this table, he suggested including anyone in my life that might have influenced me to feel that working full time right now was so important. As we parted, I remember thinking this was a crazy idea that couldn't work, but I would try it anyway.

To my surprise it worked beatifully to relieve my guilt and lessen the stress of the whole situation. When I saw him a few days later, I thanked him. My point here is that even if you think something may not work to relieve stress, have an open mind and try it. You may be surprised how helpful it can be.

Following are some stress-busting techniques for you to pick and choose from. Try the strategies that appeal most to you. But remember to be open. A suggestion you're skeptical of could end up being surprisingly helpful. By developing and practicing these techniques now, you can reduce your stress, prevent negative impacts on your health and boost your ability to manage future challenges. Take it from my friend and former colleague Dr. Amit Sood, a stress expert who has written several books on stress and happiness: "The tree does not weather a bad storm by growing deep roots the night of the rain."

Practice positive-self talk

Self-talk is the endless stream of thoughts that run through your head every day. These thoughts may be positive or negative. Some are based on logic and reason. Others may be misconceptions based on a lack of information, irrational fears or harmful beliefs.

The goal of positive self-talk is to weed out misconceptions and challenge them with self-compassion and rational, positive thoughts. Start by following one simple rule: Don't say anything to yourself that you wouldn't say to a friend or loved one. Be gentle and encouraging with yourself. If a negative thought enters your mind, evaluate it rationally and respond with statements of what is good about you.

Instead of saying, "I can't handle this," remind yourself, "Hey, I've handled bigger challenges before, and I can handle this too." Instead of telling yourself, "This is a huge disaster," try saying, "This is a big problem, but I can tackle it one step at a time." Instead of telling yourself, "I really screwed up today," say, "Everyone messes up sometimes. That's OK. It's what makes us human."

You can learn positive self-talk. The process is simple, but it takes time and practice. Throughout the day, stop and notice what you're thinking. If your thoughts are negative, counter them with a more positive perspective. Eventually, your self-talk will automatically contain less self-criticism and more self-acceptance. Your spontaneous thoughts will become more positive and rational, your confidence will grow, and your stress levels will go down.

Harness the power of optimism

Optimism can be a stress reducer and a health booster. Some research suggests that optimists may cope better with stressful situations, such as major life transitions. Many studies also show that optimists have a lower risk of heart attack and premature death.

Studies have also shown that optimism can be learned. One of the best ways to cultivate optimism is to practice daily gratitude. You can start by becoming more aware of the events, experiences and relationships that enrich your life and give it meaning.

A simple but effective habit is to practice gratitude when you first wake up in the morning or before you go to sleep at night. Instead of dwelling on your worries during these times, try thinking of three things you're grateful for. They don't have to be big things. They can be small moments that have given you pleasure: an enjoyable chat with a co-worker, an improved grade on your child's report card or a stunning sunset.

Get outside

Studies show that spending time in nature reduces stress, lowers cortisol levels, decreases blood pressure and improves well-being. For many of us the sounds, sights and smells of green spaces — such as forests, wetlands, city parks and gardens — have a powerfully calming effect. I call it "forest therapy." It's much more calming to walk in nature than to walk down a city sidewalk or even to walk in your own neighborhood.

What is the benefit? Studies have linked being outdoors with a greater reduction in inflammation in your body. If inflammation is reduced in the arteries supplying blood to your heart, then there is less chance of a heart attack; if it's reduced in the tissues of your brain, then your chances of dementia are lower; if inflammation is reduced in your colon or lungs, then there's less chance of cancer developing in those areas.

As little as 10 minutes in a green space can make a significant difference in your mood and stress level, whether you're taking a stroll or sitting down and enjoying the view. If you want to experience an even greater drop in stress, try spending 20 to 30 minutes at a time in a natural setting.

Appeal to your senses

A simple way to de-stress is to engage your senses — touch, smell, sight, taste and hearing. Hang a colorful poster or cheerful family

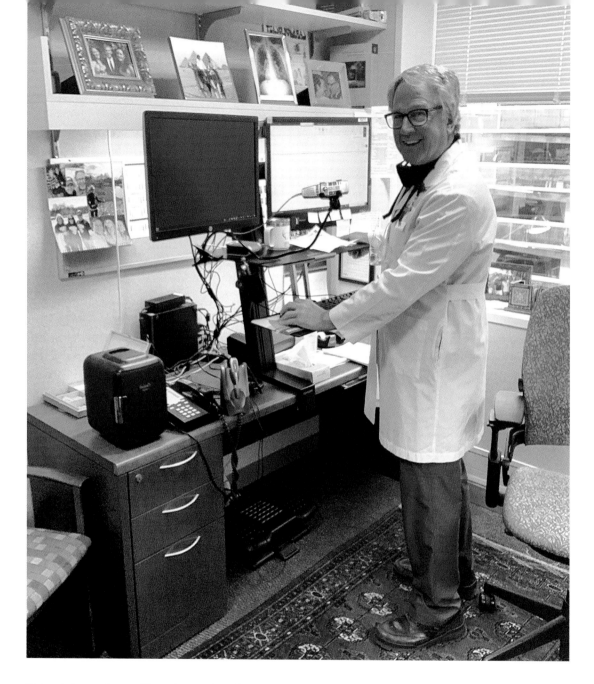

This picture of my office shows the nice rug, which has a heavy foam pad beneath it for support, and the minifridge on the corner of my desk, which has healthy snacks and foods. You cannot hear Beethoven playing in the background or smell the aromatherapy, but both are there. The pictures above my desk of my family, along with my chest X-ray with lung metastases, remind me every day how lucky I am to be here.

photo in your workspace. Listen to some peaceful music or a recording of ocean waves. Take off your shoes and notice the way the carpet or floor feels under your bare feet.

Pleasant smells can be another stress reliever. Aromatherapy, for example, uses essential oils that contain fragrant extracts from natural sources, such as leaves, flowers and fruits. Essential oils that may help you relax include lavender (which interestingly has been found to be very calming for men), frankincense, jasmine, and lemon or orange. You can infuse a space with a calming scent by placing some essential oil in a diffuser, pouring a few drops on a nearby tissue or cotton ball, or spraying some water mixed with essential oil.

I put this idea into practice a few years ago at work when we switched to a new electronic health record system, which was a major change for our institution. Talking to colleagues at other universities, I learned that the switch was a tremendous source of stress since it had to be accomplished fairly quickly while still taking care of patients. It was described as remodeling a plane while you're flying it.

To limit my stress from the switch-over, I decided to make my office a source of calm. I started to use aromatherapy in the office (smell), brought in a beautiful oriental rug (sight) with a thick cushion pad underneath it to make it more comfortable to stand on (touch), and subscribed to a music service that provided relaxing classical music (hear-ing). I even bought a mini-fridge for some healthy comfort food to snack on in the afternoon. These changes, while small, have helped me tremendously to manage my stress throughout the day, and I have noticed colleagues doing the same. Some even come into my office and say, "Can I just sit here for a few moments to relax?" to which my response is "Please — be my guest."

Help others

When you're caught up in your own worries, the last thing you may want to do is help others. But studies on helping others show that shifting the focus from yourself to other people may not only relieve stress but improve your overall health and well-being.

When our children were young, our family volunteered every Thanksgiving for over 10 years serving meals at the local Salvation Army. Our now-adult kids have commented how good they felt inside about practicing kindness and spending time in service to others. And they now see it as having a stress-reducing effect.

There are many ways to help in your community. Consider serving at a food bank or raking an elderly neighbor's lawn. Even small acts of kindness, like giving a stranger a compliment, can affect your attitude, outlook and health. Dr. Sood taught many people how important it is to practice compassion, gratitude, acceptance, meaning and forgiveness. He advises picking one trait to focus on each day.

FIND WAYS TO RELAX

Learning how to relax in the face of stress takes practice. These techniques can help you calm your body and mind.

- **Relaxed breathing.** Sit or lie in a comfortable position. Rest one hand comfortably on your abdomen and the other hand on your chest. Inhale slowly through your nose for a count of four while pushing your abdomen out. Hold your breath for a count of four. Then slowly exhale through your mouth for a count of four while pushing your abdomen in. Concentrate on breathing this way for a few minutes and become aware of the hand on your abdomen rising and falling with each breath.
- **Progressive muscle relaxation.** Sit or lie in a comfortable position and close your eyes. Allow your jaw to drop and your eyelids to be relaxed but not tightly closed. Tighten the muscles in one area of your body and hold them for a count of five. Release the tightness completely and move on to the next part of your body. Start by tensing and relaxing the muscles in your toes and progressively working your way up to your neck and head. Alternatively, you can start with your head and neck and work down to your toes.
- **Guided imagery.** Sitting or lying comfortably, start breathing slowly, regularly and deeply. Once you're more relaxed, imagine a calming place — somewhere you feel safe, happy and comfortable. Use all of your senses to notice every detail about this great place. What do you see, hear and smell? What do you feel with your hands and under your bare feet? After five or 10 minutes, rouse yourself gradually.
- **Biofeedback.** If you have a hard time relaxing, consider asking your health care provider about biofeedback. Biofeedback is a technique you can use to learn to control some of your body's functions, such as your heart rate. During biofeedback, you're connected to electrical sensors that help you receive information about your body. This feedback helps you make subtle changes in your body to reduce stress. You can receive biofeedback training in physical therapy clinics, medical centers and hospitals. A growing number of biofeedback devices and programs also are available to use at home.

A good friend of mine felt devastated after her son died because of drugs. She was uncertain how she could deal with it. Eventually, she found the best way to cope was to work at a soup kitchen providing meals to homeless young men and women, many of whom were addicted. Helping them helped her cope with the death of her son.

Take care of your body

As you've learned in previous chapters, sleep, diet and exercise are vital for your physical health. They can also impact how you cope with stress. Get proper sleep to rejuvenate your body and help you tackle the stressors of your day in a refreshed state.

Use exercise to release brain chemicals (neurotransmitters such as dopamine, serotonin, melatonin and endocannabinoids) that can leave you feeling happier, more relaxed and less anxious.

Seek out healthy meals and snacks and limit caffeine. Too much caffeinated coffee, tea or soda will increase your stress level.

Seek help

If you're struggling to cope with the stressors in your life, consider enrolling in a stress reduction class at a community or health care center. Your doctor or a mental health professional also can provide treatment options if stress is building or if you're not functioning well.

SOCIAL SUPPORT AND STRESS

While we can learn new habits to manage stress, it's hard to manage life's challenges all on our own. One of the most potent ways to reduce stress and extend our health is through our connections with others. It's important to realize this because we're living in an era when meaningful social connections seem to be dwindling while loneliness is on the rise.

Several reports produced before the COVID-19 pandemic by the health insurer Cigna revealed that a majority of Americans struggle with loneliness. Out of 20,000 people surveyed for one report, nearly half said that they regularly go a day or more without engaging in any meaningful in-person social interactions with friends, family or others.

Although people of all ages experience loneliness from time to time, Gen Zers report the highest levels of loneliness, followed by millennials and Gen Xers. Boomers and older Americans also report feelings of loneliness but at a lower rate.

We often experience these feelings when we're socially isolated, but we may also feel lonely when we're surrounded by people who don't seem to understand or connect with us.

Why social connections matter

Humans are social animals. For many thousands of years we lived in small, tightknit communities whose members were deeply interconnected. Together we shared the responsibilities of daily living, working side by side to survive.

Fast forward to today. It's likely most of us have spent entire weekends without ever leaving home. We can order food online, stream entertainment from our couches and "connect" on social media. Of necessity, the COVID-19 pandemic reinforced these habits. An unfortunate result is that a majority of us don't feel we have the social support we need to deal with the stress in our lives.

That trend may have a direct impact not only on our stress levels but also on our longevity. Studies show that social isolation and loneliness can shorten life span and increase the risk of stress-related health conditions, such as high blood pressure and heart disease.

This need for social connection is sometimes compared to that of meerkats. These small animals live in communities and one is always up on its hind legs looking around for any possible danger while the others are eating or foraging.

THE PROS AND CONS OF SOCIAL MEDIA

Engaging in chat groups, online communities and other social media can help you strengthen or maintain connections, but it's also been known to increase feelings of loneliness and isolation. Research suggests that a lot depends on how you use social media.

If you tend to visit social networking sites to compensate for weak social support, you may wind up feeling lonelier and experiencing a reduced sense of well-being. The superficial nature of "likes" or breezy responses to your online posts can leave you feeling dissatisfied or unsupported. Superficial interactions on social media can also cause us to compare ourselves with others, leading to feelings of envy and a higher risk of depression.

If, on the other hand, you interact on social media to enhance or nurture a healthy social network, your online interactions are more likely to increase your sense of connectedness, support and well-being. Checking in with close connections and newer friends can help you maintain and even strengthen those bonds, and allow you to call on their support more easily when you need it.

Like meerkats, we all need someone who's looking out for us, who "has our back," cares about us and thinks about us. This could be a spouse or relative, maybe a church group or friends at a local community center. Or it could be a pet like a dog or a cat.

One study of people who had heart attacks found that the answer to a single question asked when the heart attack happened was a predictor of survival, or death, from that event. The question was "Does anyone or anything care if you are alive?" If the answer was no, then the chance of dying from that heart attack was twofold higher.

In contrast, a robust network of social support benefits us in a variety of ways, including helping to buffer us from the negative effects of stress. Meaningful social connections, even if they're digital or from a distance, may reduce stress-related wear and tear on our bodies, promote good mental health, enhance self-esteem, encourage healthy lifestyle behaviors, and protect brain health.

Strengthening your support network

A robust social network includes a variety of people, including friends, family members, co-workers, neighbors and other acquaintances. These relationships can play a critical role in helping us through the stress of tough times, whether we've had a bad day on the job or a year filled with loss or chronic illness. Keep in mind that quality counts more than quantity. While it's good to cultivate a diverse network of people you can connect with, you also want to nurture your relationships with a few truly close

THE VALUE OF FURRY FRIENDS

Social support can come from many corners of our lives, including our pets. Living with a beloved animal has many benefits, including lowering stress and feelings of loneliness. Even brief encounters with friendly animals can give us a boost. In one study, college students who spent just 10 minutes interacting with a cat or dog experienced significantly lower cortisol levels. Being around these types of animals has also been shown to lower heart rate and blood pressure. In fact, it's been shown that if your dog develops diabetes, your risk of diabetes increases by 35%, likely because you're not walking the dog, or yourself, enough. If you don't have a pet, consider volunteering at an animal shelter. Offer to walk a neighbor's dog or offer to care for a friend's pet during an out-of-town trip.

friends and family members who will be there for you through thick and thin.

Ideally this small but dependable team of supporters can provide you with two types of support: emotional and practical. Emotional support is a compassionate best friend who's always there to listen if you need to blow off steam or shed a few tears. Practical support may be a spouse who offers to take over a household chore so you can recover from a long day at work.

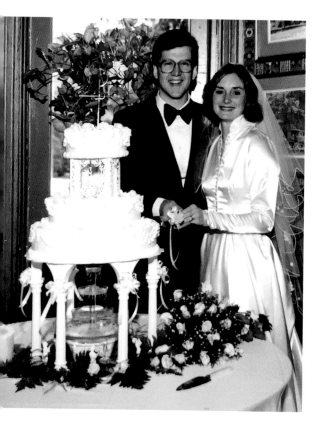

Linda and me on our wedding day. Our marriage has been a source of unbelievable happiness, tireless support and unconditional love.

Some people are good at giving both types of support, but you'll find that many people are better at one or the other — and that's OK. If you expect one person to meet all of your needs, you risk feeling disappointed or spreading that person too thin.

It's never too soon or too late to cultivate your personal support system. Here are some suggestions:

Expand your horizons If you'd like to broaden your social circle, try casting your net far and wide. Maybe you've overlooked potential friends who are already in your social network. Think through people you've interacted with — even casually — who made a positive impression. It could be someone you've encountered in your place of worship, your neighborhood, a class or a volunteering project. It might be an old friend you've lost touch with or someone you know through family connections.

If anyone stands out in your memory as someone you'd like to know better, reach out. Ask him or her to coffee or lunch. Or ask mutual friends or acquaintances to share the person's contact information or reintroduce the two of you with a text, email or in-person visit. Don't limit yourself to one strategy for meeting people. The broader your efforts, the greater your likelihood of success.

Think small Focus on little things you can do to increase your sense of connection and belonging. Start a conversation in line at the grocery store. Get to know names of the people behind the check-in counter at your fitness center. Smile and make friendly eye contact with the individuals you encounter throughout your day.

Extend and accept invitations Rather than wait for invitations to come your way, take the initiative. If your first offer isn't accepted, keep trying. A busy friend may need several gentle nudges before he or she can carve out much-needed bonding time. The same goes for a new friendship you're exploring. You may need to suggest plans a few times before you can tell if your interest in a new friend is mutual.

By the same token, be open to invitations from others. Attend family gatherings. Answer phone calls and respond to mail and email. Accept invitations to activities, even if it pushes you out of your comfort zone. You never know what doors to new friendships and acquaintances will open up.

Participate in community activities Join a fitness class through your local gym or community center. At your place of worship, take advantage of special activities and get-to-know-you events for new or existing members. Volunteer for a service project or organization in your community. Get to know people who share one of your interests or hobbies by enrolling in a class at a nearby college or community education program.

You can also look for groups or clubs that gather around an activity you enjoy. These groups are often listed in the newspaper or on community bulletin boards. There are also many websites that help you connect with new friends in your neighborhood or city.

Connect online While in-person connections are often the most sustaining, social networking sites can help you stay connected with friends and family. Online support groups may also help you get through a stressful situation. Many good sites exist for people experiencing chronic illness, the loss of a loved one, a new baby, a divorce and other life changes. Be sure to stick to reputable sites, and be cautious about arranging in-person meetings.

Give back The key to maintaining supportive adult relationships is to offer kindness and support in return. Think of your relationships as an emotional bank account. Every act of kindness and every expression of gratitude are deposits into this account, while criticism and negativity draw down the account.

Make an effort to see friends and family members regularly, and to check in with them between meetups. When you're with them, show that you care. Put down your smartphone. Ask about and listen to what's going on in their lives. If friends or family members share details of hard times or difficult experiences, be empathetic. Offer advice if they ask for it or simply be a caring listener.

"MY HEART CURRENTLY RESEMBLES THE ASHES OF MY CIGARETTES."

— English novelist and critic Virginia Woolf

CHAPTER 12

Step 5: Avoid smoking and other pollutants

It's well known that smoking can cost you a good, long life. You've probably heard many times that smoking is bad for you. For over five decades, no-smoking campaigns have spread the word about the dangers of tobacco.

The good news is that fewer Americans are smoking these days. The progress made in reducing smoking in the U.S. is one of the most important public health achievements of the past century. It came about by increasing the "friction" around smoking — raising the price and minimum age for purchasing cigarettes, putting cigarettes behind checkout counters, and decreasing their availability in vending machines.

Yet 14% of American adults still smoke. Every day, several thousand young people under the age of 18 smoke their first cigarettes.

Many of them go on to become daily smokers. In addition, many young people have taken up vaping, or using electronic cigarettes. The risks and benefits of these substitutes for traditional cigarettes are still being identified.

Meanwhile, millions of people are living with a smoking-related illness. In addition to taking a physical toll, smoking places a financial burden on the smoker, the health care system and society. Even after the warnings and education, tobacco use remains one of the most significant causes of preventable disease, disability and death in the U.S.

A BRIEF HISTORY OF TOBACCO

Before the 1880s, tobacco use in the United States was mostly chewing tobacco and cigar and pipe smoking. By the end of the century, new technology led to mass production of cigarettes that were mild in taste as well as inexpensive and convenient. During World War I, American soldiers were given cigarettes in their daily rations for relaxation and relief from pain. By the early 1920s, the use of cigarettes began to skyrocket.

Also during the 1920s, advertising broadened the appeal of smoking. Smoking had been a men's activity, but magazines and newspapers began using pictures of women smoking in fashion advertisements. This was at the same time women gained the right to vote, and cigarettes became a powerful symbol of freedom and equality. It became more acceptable for women to smoke.

At the time, doctors didn't agree about the medical consequences of smoking. In fact, tobacco use in moderation wasn't believed to be harmful. Some reports even suggested that smoking had health benefits. A doctor in Paris reported that tobacco might help prevent certain bacterial infections, and a famous mountain climber said that smoking helped his breathing at high altitudes.

In the following decades, the popularity of cigarettes continued to grow. Smoking became part of daily life in America. It was acceptable in homes, public spaces and workplaces. There were no rules or regulations, and smoke breaks were a common way to help pass the day.

It wasn't until the late 1940s and early 1950s that medical research began to show

that smoking was a cause of serious health concerns, contributing to increases in heart disease and lung cancers. While news of smoking's dangers made its way to popular magazines such as Reader's Digest, the cigarette companies countered with new filter-tip cigarettes that people assumed were safer.

But the medical evidence on the risks of smoking continued to grow, and in 1961, the major health organizations in America urged then-President John F. Kennedy to look into the harmful effects of tobacco. The result of the investigation led the Surgeon General of the United States at the time to write the first report on the dangers of tobacco in 1964. Smoking has been on the decline since then.

WHY DO PEOPLE STILL SMOKE TODAY?

Most people who smoke tobacco start when they're teenagers or young adults. For some young people, it's a way to rebel against parents and rules. Often, teens are curious, saying they "just wanted to try it." Others may feel pressure from their friends and begin smoking to fit in or feel "cool." Some may be mirroring the behavior of their parents or siblings, and others believe it's a way to relieve stress or boredom.

Media influence

Beginning with the removal of cigarette ads from television in the 1960s, there have been regulations on the marketing of tobacco that have changed and increased throughout the years. However, the media remains a big influence on smoking today. Studies show that the media affects the likelihood young people will start smoking as well as what kinds of tobacco people smoke. Tobacco companies also use price breaks and promotions to get their products seen by as many as possible.

The power of nicotine addiction

Most smokers want to quit, but tobacco use is an addiction fueled by nicotine, a powerfully addictive drug. In a matter of seconds after taking a puff of cigarette smoke, nicotine from the tobacco reaches your brain. After your brain receives the nicotine, the brain cells release dopamine. One of dopamine's effects is alertness and contentment. It may feel pleasant, like a bit of an adrenaline rush. The effects of nicotine start to wear off after several minutes, and it can leave you feeling edgy and irritable until you have another cigarette.

As you continue to smoke, your brain cells quickly change to expect the extra dopamine and your body builds up a tolerance to nicotine. You'll have to smoke more cigarettes to get the same effects. Without nicotine to deliver the dopamine your body wants, your body experiences strong cravings. Stopping smoking can cause withdrawal that includes not only physical symptoms such as headaches, dizziness and trouble sleeping but also emotional symptoms such as irritability, nervousness and depression.

The modern cigarette

In the first half of the twentieth century, cigarettes were simpler than they are now. Through the years, cigarette manufacturers have added filters, vents and flavors to cigarettes. Yet changes to cigarettes didn't make them any safer. In fact, they've become more deadly through the years. This may be because of the added chemicals and the modern design, which requires the smoker to inhale more deeply, drawing the smoke deeper into the lungs.

When the low-tar cigarette was introduced in the 1950s, the cigarette company added ammonia, which allowed for quicker absorption of nicotine. Have you ever heard of the term *freebase*, linked to drugs like cocaine? The principles are the same — you add a base like ammonia (versus an acid) to the cocaine, or the cigarette in this case, which allows it to be absorbed more quickly into the bloodstream, providing the desired addictive effects. Consequently, low-tar cigarettes were even more addictive and harmful.

In today's tobacco smoke, scientists have identified over 7,000 chemicals and chemical compounds, including radioactive materials from the fertilizers used to grow the tobacco. Many of these chemicals are poisons.

THE HARMS OF SMOKING

When you inhale tobacco smoke, the chemicals quickly travel from your lungs into your blood, reaching every organ in your body. As the chemicals get into your body, they cause inflammation in any tissue they come in contact with. We discussed inflammation earlier — it's a major underlying cause of the noncommunicable diseases we develop including cancer, heart disease and stroke. Your body's immune system, which works to fight diseases and injury, works to heal the damage, but continued smoking means your body is in a constant fight to heal itself.

A former Surgeon General's report compares smoking to spilling drain cleaner on your skin, which would cause pain and swelling. If you spill the drain cleaner on your skin repeatedly, your skin won't be able to heal. It will stay irritated. The organs in your body are made of cells similar to skin cells. When you keep smoking, the damage cannot heal, and your immune system works overtime. Research shows that this stress can lead to disease in almost any part of your body.

The poisons in tobacco smoke can pose an immediate danger — sudden blood clots, heart attacks and strokes can be brought on by tobacco smoke. Even the occasional cigarette or sitting in a smoke-filled room is enough to hurt you.

But the more years you smoke, the more you hurt your body. Smoking increases the risk of many life-threatening diseases, including cancer, emphysema and heart disease. There also are lesser known health concerns caused by smoking — tuberculosis, certain eye diseases, heartburn and problems with the immune system.

For every person who dies because of smoking, there are over two dozen people living with a serious smoking-related illness that can be ongoing and crippling.

Cancer

There are 70 different poisons in cigarette smoke that are known to cause cancer. Cancer is a serious disease in which abnormal cells grow uncontrollably, spreading throughout the body and invading other tissues. Because cells are tiny, years sometimes pass before the cancer is diagnosed.

Smoking can cause cancer almost anywhere in the body, including the:
• Blood
• Bladder
• Cervix
• Colon and rectum
• Esophagus
• Kidneys
• Liver
• Lungs
• Mouth, throat and larynx
• Pancreas
• Stomach

Smoking causes cancer by altering a cell's DNA. The DNA is the cell's "instruction manual," which controls the cell's growth and function. When the DNA is damaged, cells can begin growing abnormally.

Tobacco smoke also affects your body's ability to fight cancer. Typically, your body's immune system activates special cells to destroy the abnormal, cancerous cells. However, toxic chemicals in cigarette smoke can weaken your immune system, making it easier for the cancer cells to keep growing, dividing and spreading.

Lung disease

From the moment tobacco smoke enters your body, its poisons attack the cells that line your airways and lungs. Over time, the small, hairlike cells called cilia that clear the lungs of mucus and dirt are damaged. The lungs cannot get clear, and this can leave you with a wheeze called "smoker's cough." Also, your lungs normally stretch and expand when you breathe in and they compress when you breathe out. But years of smoking can impair this flexibility.

Smoking is the major cause of chronic obstructive pulmonary disease (COPD). COPD refers to a group of conditions that cause airflow blockages and breathing-related problems. COPD includes emphysema, chronic bronchitis and in some cases, asthma.

Heart disease and stroke

Smoking causes heart disease and stroke. Your blood vessels react almost immediately to the poisons in tobacco smoke. When the smoke is inhaled into your lungs, your blood pressure goes up and your heart rate increases as the poisons travel quickly through your blood, affecting your heart and the pathways to and from your heart.

With continued smoking, cigarettes raise your triglycerides, a type of blood fat, while lowering your "good" cholesterol. Smoking damages the lining of blood vessels (endothelium), causing thickening and narrowing of arteries. In addition, smoking increases the buildup of other fats, cholesterol, calcium and other substances in your blood vessels. Plus, it makes the blood sticky and more likely to clot, which can block blood flow to your heart and brain and cause death.

Reproductive effects

If you want to have children, smoking is a bad idea. Smoking affects not only your fertility but also the health of babies before and after they're born.

Studies show that smoking affects hormones, and it can make it difficult for women to get pregnant. During pregnancy, smoking can cause complications such as miscarriage, premature delivery and even birth defects. Mothers who smoke are also more likely to have babies with low birth weight, and there is an increased chance of sudden infant death syndrome.

For men, smoking is a cause of erectile dysfunction. Men with erectile dysfunction can't have or maintain an erection necessary for sexual performance. Studies have shown that smoking can also damage the DNA in men's sperm, which might affect the ability to father a child. It might also cause miscarriages and birth defects.

Other harmful effects

Other major health concerns from smoking include the increased risk of:

- Type 2 diabetes, which can lead to amputation, blindness and kidney failure.
- Autoimmune issues, such as rheumatoid arthritis, in which the body attacks healthy cells, causing joint pain and swelling.
- Eye diseases, including age-related macular degeneration and cataracts.
- Digestive problems that include heartburn (acid reflux), stomach ulcers and Crohn's disease.

HOW TO QUIT SMOKING

No matter how long you've been smoking, quitting will improve your health in moments (see page 170). Quitting can be difficult, but there are proven treatments and strategies to help you be successful.

Most people find that a combination of approaches works best. In particular, a combination of counseling and medication has shown to be the most effective. Don't get discouraged as you try to quit. Most people need several tries to successfully quit.

Medications

Medications can more than double your chances of quitting smoking. They help lessen the intensity of nicotine withdrawal and help quiet your urge to smoke. While nicotine withdrawal doesn't pose any health risks, it can be uncomfortable and is usually the worst in the first week.

Medicines include nicotine replacement therapies (patches, gum, lozenges or prescription-only inhalers and nasal spray). These give you a small amount of nicotine to help with withdrawal and cravings, without the dangerous chemicals in cigarette smoke. Using a combination of therapies helps increase your chances of quitting. For example, combining a long-acting patch with a shorter-acting gum or lozenge is more effective than using a single form.

Prescription medicines such as varenicline and bupropion also can help reduce withdrawal symptoms and cravings.

Counseling

Counseling can help increase your chances of quitting successfully. It can help you learn how to cope with the withdrawal, cravings, stress, mood changes and other challenges that come with quitting tobacco.

Counseling is available in a variety of ways, including one on one with a health care professional or in a support group. There are also web-based and text messaging programs to offer support.

Find help over the phone by calling 800-QUIT-NOW, where you can talk to a trained counselor and receive practical information as well as referrals to other resources. You also can visit *www.BecomeAnEx.org* or call the Mayo Clinic Nicotine Dependence Center at 800-344-5984.

Other practical, proven steps to success include the following:
- Set a specific quit date.
- Talk to a doctor, nurse, pharmacist or other health care provider. He or she can talk to you about tools to help you reach your goals safely and effectively.
- Seek out a support network. Ask family, friends and ex-smokers for their support, or join a local or online support group.
- Know what triggers your desire to use tobacco, and change your daily routines to avoid those situations.
- Practice coping strategies such as deep breathing, meditation or exercise to take your mind off smoking.
- Think positively. Remind yourself that you're healthier and stronger living life tobacco free.

JUST AS HARMFUL AS SMOKING

Smoking cigarettes clearly is harmful. But there are other ways that pollutants can enter your body and cause harm.

Secondhand smoke

Secondhand smoke is the smoke that comes from the burning end of a cigarette, cigar or pipe. It also includes the smoke that smokers breathe out. Research shows that when you inhale secondhand smoke, you're exposed to the same poisonous, cancer-caus-ing chemicals that smokers are. There's no safe level of secondhand smoke, and even being around secondhand smoke for a short period of time can be dangerous.

Ross Rebagliati is a reminder of the power of secondhand smoke. He won the snowboarding gold medal for Canada at the Olympics in 1998. Yet he was stripped of his medal after a post-race drug test in which he tested positive for tetrahydrocannabinol (THC), the active ingredient in marijuana. He insisted that he had not smoked marijuana, but he'd spent time with friends prior to the race who were smoking. His secondhand inhalation of the smoke was enough for him to test positive. (After a review by Olympic officials, his medal was returned to him.)

You can protect yourself from secondhand smoke by:
- Not allowing smoking in your home, in your car or around your children.
- Keeping smoke outside. It isn't enough to open windows or use air-cleaning devices. It can take three hours for smoke to clear from a room.
- Avoiding areas and public places where people smoke.

Thirdhand smoke

A smoker doesn't even have to light up to put those in the vicinity at risk. While secondhand smoke is smoke you inhale from someone else's cigarette, thirdhand smoke is toxic residue that settles on clothes, hair, walls and other surfaces. If you touch it or smell it, you can absorb it.

REWARDS OF QUITTING TOBACCO

Within 20 minutes after you smoke that last cigarette, your body begins a series of healthy changes. These beneficial changes make a difference for years.

20 MINUTES AFTER QUITTING — Heart rate and blood pressure drops.

12 HOURS AFTER QUITTING — Carbon monoxide blood level drops to normal.

2 WEEKS TO 3 MONTHS AFTER QUITTING — Coughing and shortness of breath decrease. Blood circulation improves.

1 YEAR AFTER QUITTING — Added risk of coronary artery disease is half that of a smoker's. Risk of heart attack has decreased significantly.

5 YEARS AFTER QUITTING — Risk of a stroke is reduced to that of someone who doesn't smoke.

10 YEARS AFTER QUITTING — Chance of dying of lung cancer is about half that of a smoker's. Risk of cancers of the mouth, throat, esophagus, bladder, kidney and pancreas decrease.

15 YEARS AFTER QUITTING — Risk of coronary artery disease is that of a non-smoker.

Young children, especially those whose parents are smokers, are particularly at risk of exposure to thirdhand smoke. Even if you smoke outside, the smoke clings to your clothes and hair. When your child sits on your lap and inhales the smoke aroma and is exposed to the smoke on your clothes, this qualifies as thirdhand smoke exposure. Although direct health effects from thirdhand smoke haven't been established, many of the substances that are left on surfaces are known cancer-causing toxins. There's concern about long-term exposure to these chemicals, even if it's at low levels.

The lasting effects of thirdhand smoke may linger in homes for months or even years after smoking has stopped. To reduce thirdhand smoke, you may need to clean and repaint or replace drywall, carpets or other affected materials. You may want to ask before buying or renting a home about prior smoking in the home.

Vaping

Vaping is the use of e-cigarettes and other electronic vaping devices. The devices are sometimes called e-cigs, e-hookahs, mods, vape pens, vapes, tank systems and electronic nicotine delivery systems (ENDS). If you use or have considered using e-cigarettes, you might wonder if they're really a safer or healthier option or if they can help you quit smoking.

Some e-cigarettes resemble traditional cigarettes, cigars or pipes, and some look like

other everyday items such as highlighters, remote controls and pens. E-cigarettes are battery-operated devices that can be disposable or refillable. Most use a cartridge or pod to hold liquid, also called e-liquid or e-juice. The device heats the liquid to make the aerosol, which users inhale into their lungs.

The liquid typically contains nicotine, flavorings and other chemicals to make the aerosol. However, some liquids can also contain harmful substances such as THC.

Is it safe? The easy-to-get and easy-to-use vaping devices are often seen as harmless, but there have been cases of lung injury tied to vaping. Most of the injuries have involved products containing THC. The Centers for Disease Control and Prevention (CDC) and the Food and Drug Administration (FDA) recommend that people not use vaping products that contain THC. If you vape, watch for symptoms like coughing, shortness of breath and chest pain. Seek medical attention if you're concerned about your health.

E-cigarettes containing nicotine aren't considered safe for teenagers, young adults or pregnant women. Nicotine can harm brain development in children and young adults into their early twenties and is toxic to developing fetuses. Children and adults have also been poisoned by swallowing, breathing or absorbing e-cigarette liquid through their skin or eyes. The aerosol that users breathe and exhale from the devices can contain harmful and potentially harmful substances.

E-cigarette use also poses the risk of nicotine addiction. Addiction could lead to long-term use of e-cigarettes, the effects of which aren't known, or to the use of traditional cigarettes. Research has shown that teen use of e-cigarettes is on the rise and associated with increased future use of traditional cigarettes.

Will it help me quit smoking? E-cigarettes aren't approved by the FDA as a quit aid. Studies to test whether e-cigarettes can help people stop using tobacco have had inconsistent results. Limited research suggests that using e-cigarettes containing nicotine to quit smoking can be effective when accompanied by face-to-face support. But more evidence is needed to prove the safety and effectiveness of e-cigarettes for smoking cessation, particularly over the long term.

So far, e-cigarettes haven't been proved to be safe, nor are they necessarily more effective in helping people stop smoking than the FDA-approved medicines that have undergone extensive safety testing.

Because of these concerns, at Mayo Clinic we don't recommend the use of e-cigarettes. If you do use e-cigarettes to quit smoking, remember that your goal is to completely quit using all tobacco products. Also, the dual use of e-cigarettes containing nicotine and traditional cigarettes is strongly discouraged.

Cigars

While cigarettes are wrapped in paper, cigars are wrapped in tobacco and filled with a type of fermented tobacco. This gives the cigars a different taste and smell from cigarettes. Today's cigars come in different sizes, sometimes with filters and flavoring. Larger cigars weren't traditionally inhaled, but some of today's cigar companies are changing the way cigars are made so that the smoke is easier to inhale.

Cigars lost popularity in the 1920s when cigarettes became more available. Cigar smoking became an activity that most people associated with older men. But with popular magazines centered around cigar smoking and the modern trend of neighborhood cigar bars, cigar smoking has increased and is viewed by many as sophisticated and less dangerous than smoking cigarettes.

However, the belief that cigars are less dangerous than cigarettes is a myth. A large cigar can contain as much nicotine as a pack of cigarettes. Cigars contain the same cancer-causing ingredients found in cigarettes and aren't a safe alternative to cigarettes.

Air quality

An often overlooked but important part of your health is the quality of the air you breathe. Air pollution is a leading environmental risk factor around the world, causing millions of deaths worldwide. While the U.S. has made great strides since the 1990s toward improving outdoor air quality, challenges remain. Your awareness and understanding of the risks can help protect you and your loved ones.

When it comes to air quality, the most important contributor to your health risk is particle pollution, also called particulate matter or PM. PM is the tiny particles, or pieces, of solids or liquids that are in the air.

Particle pollution comes from different sources. Forest fires, road dust, electrical power plants, industrial facilities, cars and trucks give off particles directly. Other sources responsible for PM, such as coal-fired power plants and exhaust from cars and trucks, give off gases that react with sunlight and water to form particles.

Breathing in particle pollution can have harmful consequences for your health. The bigger particles from dust around farms, dry riverbeds, construction sites and mines can irritate your eyes, nose and throat. The smaller particles, less than 1/30 the width of a human hair, are more dangerous to your health. They can get deep into your lungs, where they can affect the heart, blood vessels and lungs.

Particle pollution can affect anyone, but it bothers some people more than others. People with heart disease or lung disease, including asthma, are most likely to experience health effects. Older adults, babies and children also are at risk. In addition, people exposed to PM over a long period of time have a higher risk of heart and lung problems.

The good news is that the U.S. has low particle pollution. In addition, the Environmental Protection Agency (EPA) has a website called AirNow, which shows you the air quality around the country. It measures PM, as well as ground-level ozone, which is a harmful pollutant and main ingredient in smog. AirNow lets you know when air pollution is likely to reach levels that could put your health at risk. You can use it before you plan your daily activities: *www.airnow.gov.*

POSITIVE TRENDS

Cigarette smoking has reached an all-time low among adults in the United States. This tremendous achievement is the result of decadeslong work to raise awareness, implement public health policies and provide effective, proven ways to quit. The efforts have reduced smoking in adults by over two-thirds since the 1960s.

What more can be done?

The FDA is committed to continuing the trend. It's working to make cigarettes minimally or nonaddictive and there's support for the development of new nicotine replacement therapies. At the same time, the work to protect kids from the dangers of tobacco and vaping is ongoing.

But the reality remains — cigarette smoking is one of the leading preventable causes of death and disease in the United States. The work to end the epidemic of tobacco-related diseases is not finished. And a good, long life depends on it.

DRINKING ALCOHOL HAS BENEFITS
AND RISKS. MODERATION IS KEY.

CHAPTER 13

Step 6: Be thoughtful about alcohol

A good, long life is full of moments, both big and small, that we recognize and celebrate — a much-anticipated wedding, the closing of an important business deal, the end of a long work week. For thousands of years, all around the world, people have marked these moments by raising a glass and sharing a drink.

In fact, alcohol has been made by humans for centuries. Long ago it was felt to be a healthier option to drink than water because of its antimicrobial properties, making it a better way to quench thirst.

Today, alcohol remains a big part of our culture. Billions of dollars are spent in our economy on the consumption of alcohol. Also, having a drink is at the center of many of our social functions. From the neighborhood bar to the shared bottle of wine at a family dinner, people come together over a drink to celebrate, relax and bond.

Alcoholic beverages are unique because they're considered both a food and a drug. As a food, it gives you calories and refreshment, but as a drug, it can be intoxicating and can affect your body's systems, including mood and coordination. While you can experience alcohol as a source of pleasure and release, in excess it's known for its dangers to health and society.

For researchers, drinking alcohol is one of the most challenging lifestyle factors to study, especially over long periods of time. It's difficult to separate the effects of drinking on your health from all the other parts of your life, such as your sex, age, genes, stress levels, sleep habits, diet or exercise routine.

Still, some studies have shown that drinking a small amount of alcohol may be beneficial to your heart. To help you make good decisions about your health and well-being, this chapter will take a close look at the recommended guidelines, the potential benefits and the risks of drinking alcohol.

WHAT'S THE DIFFERENCE BETWEEN MODERATE AND HEAVY DRINKING?

Before you examine the risks and benefits of drinking alcohol, it's important to understand the difference between moderate and heavy drinking.

If you're a healthy adult and you're going to drink, it's recommended that you drink in moderation. Drinking in moderation is associated with a relatively low risk for alcohol problems. For a healthy adult woman, moderation generally means no more than one drink a day and fewer than seven drinks in a week. For healthy adult men, guidelines recommend drinking no more than two drinks a day and fewer than 14 drinks a week.

Drinking more than the moderate drinking guidelines, however, can be harmful. Whether on a single occasion or over time, heavy drinking is risky. It's considered heavy drinking for a woman to consume eight or more drinks a week or for a man to have 15 or more drinks a week. Included in the definition of heavy drinking is binge drinking, which is consuming four or more drinks for a woman or five or more drinks for a man on an occasion.

And for some people, there's no safe level of alcohol use. For example, check with your doctor before drinking if:

- You're taking certain over-the-counter or prescription medicines that may interact with alcohol.
- You've been diagnosed with alcoholism or alcohol addiction, or you have a strong family history of alcoholism.
- You're pregnant or trying to get pregnant.
- You've had a hemorrhagic stroke (when a blood vessel in your brain leaks or ruptures).
- You have liver or pancreatic disease.
- You've had certain types of cancer, such as breast cancer.
- You have heart failure or you've been told you have a weak heart.

ARE THERE BENEFITS TO DRINKING IN MODERATION?

Can drinking alcohol actually have benefits for your health? The answer brings us to something called the "U-shaped" curve that researchers have often observed when it comes to alcohol (see page 178). Drinking no alcohol and drinking too much both are associated with increased mortality and morbidity (a word doctors use for disease).

But an adult having a small amount can actually derive health benefits. Studies show that a total daily amount of 3 ounces of wine for women and 5 ounces for men is probably the best amount to help you reach the bottom of the U-shaped curve, which represents the lowest chance of dying.

Why alcohol in small amounts appears to be beneficial isn't exactly known. Perhaps it relates to alcohol's relaxing effects, or the fact that it lowers your blood pressure by temporarily enlarging your arteries. Remember, the bigger the pipe, the lower the pressure.

Does it matter what you drink? Probably not. What matters more is how much you drink. Ethyl alcohol, which is the type of alcohol found in wine, beer or hard liquor, is the same no matter what it's brewed from. Ethyl alcohol is what yeast molecules produce when they ingest carbohydrates (fermentation process). Traditionally, grapes render wine, barley and malt give us beer, and a variety of carbs give us bourbon (from corn), gin (juniper berries) or vodka (potatoes).

Some studies show that compared to no drinking and heavy drinking, there may be some benefits for drinking alcohol in moderation, such as:

- Reducing your risk of developing and dying of heart disease
- Possibly reducing your risk of an ischemic stroke (when the arteries to your brain become narrowed or blocked, causing severely reduced blood flow)
- Possibly reducing your risk of diabetes

However, other researchers question these results. Almost all studies of lifestyle, including diet, exercise, caffeine and alcohol, rely on personal recall of habits over many years. These studies may indicate an association between two things, but not necessarily that one causes the other. It may be that adults who are in good health engage in more social activities and enjoy moderate amounts of alcohol, but that the alcohol has nothing to do with making them healthier.

▶ ONE DRINK IS DEFINED AS:

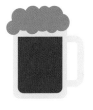

BEER
12 oz., 5% alcohol

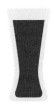

MALT LIQUOR
8 oz., 7% alcohol

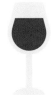

WINE
5 oz., 12% alcohol

DISTILLED SPIRITS
1.5 oz., 40% alcohol

Each drink contains 14 grams of alcohol.

So, experts are hesitant to promote the potential benefits of alcohol. There's little agreement on how much drinking is too much to receive any benefit. In addition, the balance between risk and benefit can vary with different age groups and groups of people. The benefit of drinking moderately must also be balanced against the effect of alcohol on other disorders, such as liver problems and cancer. For example, for a young woman who has a low risk of heart disease, the increased risk related to alcohol

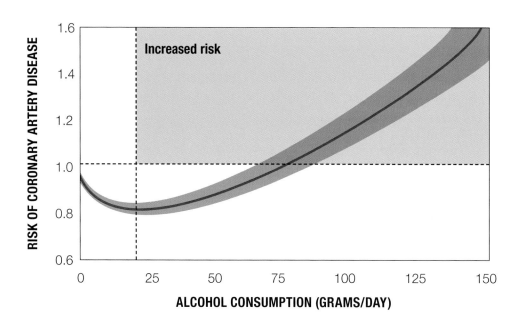

ALCOHOL'S U-SHAPED CURVE

Although the research remains controversial, most studies have found that light to moderate alcohol consumption may be protective of heart health. Heavy alcohol consumption, on the other hand, increases the risk of heart disease and premature death. This creates a relationship that looks like a U- or J-shaped curve.

Source: *Journal of Internal Medicine.* 2015;278:238.

intake and breast cancer might outweigh any potential heart benefits.

THE COSTS OF HEAVY DRINKING

Health risks increase with the amount of alcohol you drink. Drinking too much can affect your health in the short and long term.

Short-term health risks

Heavy drinking has the near-term effect of increasing your risk of:

- **Injuries.** Drinking too much increases the risk of accidental injuries from motor vehicle crashes, falls, drownings and burns.
- **Violence.** It also increases the risk of violence, including homicide, suicide, sexual assault and domestic violence.
- **Poisonings.** Excessive drinking can lead to alcohol poisoning, which is potentially fatal and happens by drinking large amounts of alcohol in a short period of time. Alcohol use also contributes to poisonings and overdoses from other substances, including opioids.
- **Sexually transmitted infections and unintended pregnancy.** Those who binge drink are more likely to have unprotected sex and multiple sex partners, increasing the risk of sexually transmitted infections and unintended pregnancy.
- **Birth defects.** Heavy alcohol use during pregnancy can cause fetal alcohol spectrum disorders, or FASD, which can result in lifelong physical, mental and behavioral problems.

Long-term health risks

Over time, heavy drinking can have serious consequences. It's a leading cause of preventable death in the U.S. In fact, along with tobacco use, poor nutrition and lack of exercise, heavy drinking is considered a main risk factor for preventable, chronic disease. Heavy drinking is known to cause the following:

- **Brain damage.** If you drink large amounts of alcohol over long periods of time, you run the risk of developing changes in the brain. Damage may be a result of the direct effects of alcohol on the brain, or it may result indirectly, from poor overall health or severe liver disease. Problems can affect both your memory and your mental health.
- **High blood pressure.** When alcohol is metabolized by the body, one of the compounds produced is acetaldehyde, which sounds like formaldehyde. And acetaldehyde's effects on our arteries is similar to formaldehyde — it "pickles" them, or makes the arteries stiff and raises blood pressure every time the heart beats. The heart beats an average of 100,000 times a day, so even small increases in blood pressure make more work for the heart with every beat, magnifying the heart's workload tremendously.
- **Heart problems.** Heavy drinking and binge drinking can damage your heart. It can cause a stretching and drooping of the heart muscle, called cardiomyopathy, as well as an irregular heartbeat, high blood pressure, heart failure or a stroke. Alcohol at any dose can cause irregular

WHEN THE BRAKES GO OUT: ALCOHOL USE DISORDER

A risk of drinking alcohol is its potential to produce dependence. This can lead to AUD, or alcohol use disorder. AUD includes a level of drinking that's sometimes called alcoholism. It's a pattern of alcohol use that involves difficulty controlling your drinking, being preoccupied with alcohol, continuing to use alcohol even when it causes problems, having to drink more to get the same effect, or having withdrawal symptoms when you rapidly decrease or stop drinking. If your pattern of drinking results in repeated distress and problems functioning in your daily life, you likely have alcohol use disorder.

AUD can range from mild to severe. However, even a mild disorder can escalate and lead to serious problems, so early treatment is important. If you feel that you sometimes drink too much alcohol, or your drinking is causing problems, or your family is concerned about your drinking, talk with your doctor. Other ways to get help include talking with a mental health professional or seeking help from a support group such as Alcoholics Anonymous or a similar type of self-help group.

heartbeats due to its direct toxicity on the heart muscle and electrical conduction system.

- **Liver disease.** Alcohol is the leading cause of liver disease. Your liver does the work of breaking down the alcohol during the digestive process. Heavy drinking takes a toll on the liver, and it can lead to swelling and a variety of problems, including increased fat in the liver (hepatic steatosis), inflammation of the liver (alcoholic hepatitis), and over time, irreversible destruction and scarring of liver tissue (cirrhosis).
- **Digestive problems.** Heavy drinking can result in inflammation of the stom-

ach lining and pancreas, as well as stomach and esophageal ulcers. It can also interfere with absorption of vitamins and other nutrients.
- **Cancer.** There's strong evidence of a connection between drinking alcohol and several types of cancer, including head and neck, esophageal, colorectal, liver, and breast cancer. The evidence suggests that the more you drink, the higher the risk. The U.S. Department of Health and Human Services lists alcohol as a known cancer-causing substance (carcinogen).
- **Sexual function and menstrual issues.** Excessive drinking can cause erectile

dysfunction in men. In women, it can interrupt menstruation.

- **Weakened immune system.** Drinking too much can weaken your immune system, making your body an easier target for disease. Heavy drinkers are vulnerable to infections like pneumonia and tuberculosis. If you binge drink, it slows your body's ability to ward off infections, even 24 hours after getting drunk.

THE THREE A'S

If alcohol is a part of your diet, be intentional about when and how you choose to drink. Obviously, we want to avoid drinking too much. But I also like to keep in mind the three "A's" that detract from a healthy and thoughtful approach to alcohol:

- **Automatic drinking.** By this, I mean drinking out of habit, without thinking. For some of us, approaching the end of the workday can trigger the desire for a drink. One recommendation I often make is to alternate each drink with something nonalcoholic, such as sparkling water, in the same glass. This typically cuts the amount of alcohol you consume in half. If you're thirsty, have a nonalcoholic drink nearby to quench your thirst rather than alcohol. If you drink for the taste, say a nice wine, keep in mind that we only have 2,000 to 4,000 taste buds in our mouths and it only takes about 20 drops to saturate them. Anything more is wasted in terms of flavor. So when drinking alcohol for the flavor, it's best to sip, not gulp.
- **Adulterated drinking.** I think of adulterated drinking as involving drinks with lots of ingredients. A cocktail or mixed drink is a fun way to celebrate, but be aware that these drinks often come loaded with even more calories than alcohol already brings to the table. Drinking them habitually can contribute to unnecessary weight gain. Some drinks also contain added substances and chemicals that aren't healthy.
- **Addictive drinking.** This kind of drinking occurs when we've developed a dependency on alcohol, whether it be a chemical or emotional dependency, or even a mix of both. Addictive drinking is problematic because we lose control of our intake. If we're addicted to alcohol, we can't get by without it, and that's definitely not healthy. At that point, it's time to get professional help.

If you're concerned that you may be drinking too much, try cutting back to only one drink a day for a month — if you have trouble staying at that level, you likely have a problem and should seek help.

Drinking alcohol isn't risk-free. If you don't drink alcohol, don't start because of potential health benefits. However, if you drink a light to moderate amount and you're healthy, you can probably continue as long as you drink responsibly.

JUST AS OUR DAILY CHOICES CAN LEAD US TO GAIN WEIGHT OVER TIME, SO TOO CAN OUR CHOICES HELP US UNDO THAT GAIN.

CHAPTER 14

The (un)importance of weight

Obesity is a major health problem in the United States. Two-thirds of the adult population is overweight, and 1 in 3 adults is considered obese. Childhood obesity is at an all-time high.

With the easy availability of calorie-dense foods, the bombardment by commercial messages urging you to eat, and the prevalence of sedentary work and leisure activities, it's easy to pack on pounds.

After a certain point, body fat can interfere with your health. The more your weight increases, the more problems you'll face in staying healthy and living longer.

Health experts generally agree that carrying a lot of extra weight on your body can be harmful to your health. In clinical research studies, obesity — technically defined as having a body mass index (BMI) over 30 — has been repeatedly associated with an increased risk of heart disease, stroke, diabetes, certain cancers, digestive and liver problems, infertility, erectile dysfunction, sleep apnea and osteoarthritis. In fact, it's been connected to almost all of the modern illnesses that plague us. It's also linked to a higher rate of premature death.

A healthy weight is important to a good, long life. But you can achieve it without necessarily focusing on weight loss to the exclusion of all else. All of the steps outlined in the preceding chapters collectively contribute to achieving and maintaining a healthy weight. If you focus on improving your habits in terms of diet, exercise, sleep, stress management, social support and alcohol intake, your weight will likely improve, as well.

IS YOUR WEIGHT HEALTHY?

A combination of several measurements in addition to your medical history can give you an idea of whether it would be beneficial to lose a few pounds. Even a small reduction in weight can reduce your risk of heart disease, diabetes and more.

Body mass index

In the 19th century, the Belgian mathematician, astronomer and statistician Adolphe Quetelet developed the Quetelet Index, a measurement that took a person's weight in kilograms and divided it by height in meters squared to determine whether a person's body weight was "average." This system of considering body weight in relation to height was revisited years later, when insurance actuaries started noticing that their overweight policyholders had increased mortality, and researchers started taking a closer look at the relationship of weight and heart disease. Today we call this measurement body mass index (BMI).

An easy way to determine your BMI is to weigh yourself and have your height measured. Then determine your BMI by using the chart on page 198.

RISING RATES OF PREDIABETES IN THE U.S.

According to estimates from the Centers for Disease Control and Prevention, 86 million people have prediabetes in the United States but only 9 million are actually aware that they have it. The current march toward diabetes is almost inevitable, as you can see from the numbers. Much of this trend relates to excess weight.

Who has prediabetes in the U.S.?

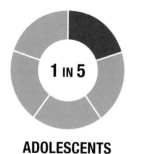

ADOLESCENTS
(ages 12-18)

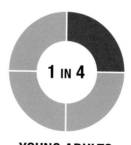

YOUNG ADULTS
(ages 19-34)

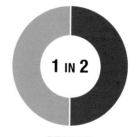

ADULTS
(ages 35 and older)

Based on Centers for Disease Control and Prevention

BMI ranges aren't exact categories of healthy and unhealthy weights, but they can give you an estimate of where you fall. A BMI of 18.5 to 24.9 is considered healthy. If your BMI falls within this range, there's generally little health advantage to your losing weight. A BMI of 25 to 29.9 suggests that you're overweight. If you have a BMI of 30 or more, you're considered obese.

The further your BMI is above the healthy range, the higher your weight-related health risks. If your BMI is 25 or more, losing weight may improve your health and reduce your risk of weight-related diseases. If your BMI falls below 18.5, you're probably underweight and may need to find ways to increase your calorie intake.

Drawbacks How accurate is BMI at predicting development of disease? BMI can't tell the difference between things that influence weight, such as bone density, muscle mass and body fat. For example, a very muscular athlete or bodybuilder might be considered obese because he or she is carrying a lot of muscle weight and thus a higher BMI.

On the other hand, BMI may not always reflect the amount of body fat a person carries. As we age, our muscle mass tends to dip lower as our fat mass inches upward. Our BMI may not change, but we might have more of an unhealthy ratio of muscle to fat. A 2019 study published in *JAMA Oncology*, for example, found that postmenopausal women with a normal BMI but higher levels of body fat had an increased risk of developing invasive breast cancer. In other words, someone with a "healthy" weight could still have unhealthy levels of body fat and all of the problems that come with it.

Waist circumference

It also matters where you carry your weight. Some people carry it primarily around their waists — excess belly fat. The trouble with belly fat is that it's not limited to the extra layer of padding located just below the skin (subcutaneous fat). It also includes visceral fat — which lies deep inside your abdomen, surrounding your internal organs.

Increased visceral fat puts you at higher risk of heart disease, diabetes, sleep apnea, high blood pressure, erectile dysfunction and some cancers, even if your BMI is about right. If your BMI is 25 or higher and your waist circumference exceeds healthy guidelines, the risk is even greater. How body fat is distributed begins with genetics, but it's also influenced by age and behavior.

Many women notice an increase in belly fat as they get older — even if they aren't gaining weight. This is likely due to a decreasing level of estrogen, which appears to influence how fat is distributed in the body.

Drinking excess alcohol can contribute to belly fat or a "beer belly," but beer alone isn't to blame. Drinking too much alcohol of any kind can cause weight gain, because alcohol contains calories in the form of processed carbohydrates.

Your waist circumference measurement can tell you whether you have too much belly fat (see page 199 for details on measuring your waist). A waist measurement of 35 inches or more for women, or 40 inches or more for men, is associated with higher health risks. In general, the smaller the waist measurement, the lower the health risks.

Waist-to-hip ratio

Another measure that's fairly accurate at predicting future disease development is the waist-to-hip ratio (WHR). Your health care provider can measure your WHR, or you can do it on your own (see page 199).

According to the World Health Organization, a healthy waist-to-hip ratio is 0.9 or less for men and 0.85 or less for women. For both men and women, a WHR of 1.0 or higher increases the risk of heart disease and other conditions that are linked to being overweight.

Compared with waist circumference and BMI, waist-to-hip ratio has been found to be a better predictor of mortality in people over 75. A study that spanned all continents in the world found that when obesity was defined using WHR instead of BMI, the proportion of people found to be at risk of heart attack worldwide increased threefold.

Measurement of body fat percentage is probably a more accurate measure of relative weight but difficult to do since it requires sophisticated medical equipment. The advantage of waist-to-hip ratio relative to BMI and waist circumference is that it takes into account the differences inherent in body structure. Thus, it's possible for two women to have a very different BMI but the same WHR, or to have the same BMI but a very different WHR.

Medical history

Your medical history can provide additional information about your health and how it relates to your weight:

- Do you have high blood pressure, diabetes, heart disease, sleep apnea, erectile dysfunction, osteoarthritis or abnormal blood fats (cholesterol and triglycerides)?
- Have you gained at least 10 pounds as an adult?
- Do you smoke cigarettes, overeat, have more than two alcoholic drinks a day or lead an inactive lifestyle?

Assessing your weight

If you answered yes to any of the medical history questions, you're likely to benefit from weight loss if you're overweight or obese. If your weight falls into the obese category, even losing just a few pounds may improve your health. A modest reduction in weight — 3% to 10% of your total weight — can improve many health conditions associated with excess weight. These include diabetes, high blood pressure, high cholesterol and sleep apnea. If your extra weight is mostly around your waist, taking just 2 inches off your waist may reduce your blood pressure and lower your risk of many diseases.

CAN GOING ON A DIET HELP YOU LOSE WEIGHT?

Every day, any given number of people around the world go on some form of a modified diet in an attempt to lose weight. Lured by the promise of rapid weight loss or a deep cleanse from ingested toxins, we hope against hope that this time our efforts will succeed and we will miraculously drop those pounds.

Over the years, our desire to be slim has fed an entire industry of diet programs, ranging from magic single ingredients to complex menus and eating plans. But our collective weight has only gone up (see the graph on page 188). Overweight and obesity continue on a relentless rise in America, as well as other places around the globe.

Why is this? For one thing, temporary diets rarely lead to long-term weight loss. Analyses of various popular eating trends show that although some may lead to weight loss in the first six months, by the end of a year any pounds shed have almost always been regained. Generally, the more rapid the initial weight loss, the greater and more rapid the subsequent weight gain.

Consumers aren't the only ones attracted to popular diets. Medical researchers and scientists, keen to find a way to fight obesity, have studied various weight-loss plans to see if they might offer an effective treatment for obesity. Two diets that have received quite a bit of medical attention include:

Low-carb diets Low-carb diets, which steer clear of carbohydrates in favor of protein and fats, have taken America by storm. A number of studies have shown that this type of eating regimen can promote weight loss, especially if you reduce your calorie intake from refined carbohydrates, such as added sugar and ultraprocessed foods.

A lot of low-carb eating plans, however, replace important sources of fiber (such as whole-grain foods and beans) with protein sources such as meat and bacon. And as we know, these can cause systemic inflammation in the body.

The truth is, you don't want to eat too few or too many carbohydrates. Based on research, the sweet spot for carb consumption is about 50% of your total calories, keeping in mind you want healthy carbs, such as those found in whole grains, vegetables, fruits, beans and legumes.

So despite the low-carb eating plan's ability to promote weight loss, following a meat-based, low-carb diet isn't all that great for your health. If you're getting a hamburger and throwing away the bun, you may find you lose weight in the short term, but this isn't doing much to lower your risk of heart disease in the long run. In fact, studies show that a diet low in carbs and rich in saturated animal fat actually increases your risk of heart attack and shortens your life span.

The (un)importance of weight   187

OBESITY RATES AND DIET TRENDS
UNITED STATES, ADULTS 20-74

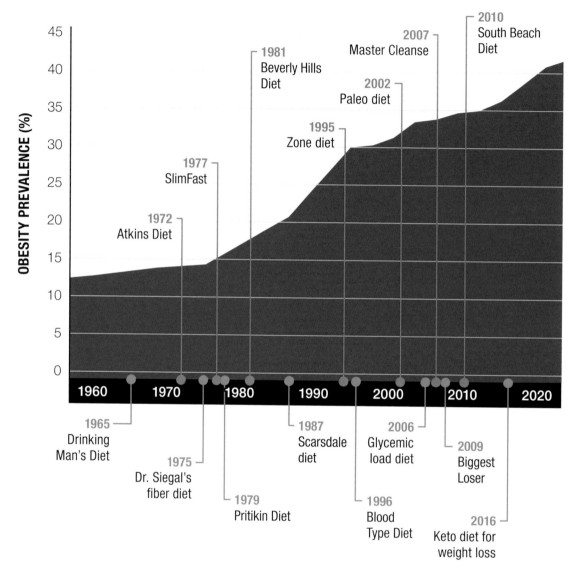

Popular diet trends over the last half-century have failed to curb obesity rates in the U.S.

Based on National Health and Nutrition Examination Survey; Library of Congress; PubMed

Time-restricted diets Some research shows that time-related patterns of eating, such as time-restricted eating and intermittent fasting, may promote weight loss. These patterns involve eating only during specific hours or certain days. You may see these referred to as "alternate-day fasting" or by popular diet names such as the 5:2 diet (eat normally for five days, restrict calories to 500 or so the other two days of the week) or the 11-7 diet (eat only between the hours of 11 a.m. and 7 p.m.).

The structure of these diets isn't exactly revolutionary. If food supplies were scarce long ago, our prehistoric ancestors might have had to go days before their next meal. The human body is built to withstand this by using its ability to switch energy sources.

During fasting periods, our bodies switch from burning liver-derived energy to burning energy derived from fat cells (ketones). In general, ketones start rising after about eight to 12 hours of fasting, a condition called ketosis. Using this alternate source of fuel is supposed to improve blood sugar regulation, suppress inflammation, repair damaged cells and aid in weight loss. Also, it helps that when you go into ketosis, you tend to get a little nauseated and lose your appetite.

And yet, studies examining time-restricted eating show that it may not be any better than other diets in achieving long-term weight loss. Why? Because any dietary pattern that you can't follow for the rest of your life won't produce long-term weight loss.

The bottom line is that there are many factors that affect body weight and that managing weight is much more complex than removing this food or that food or manipulating eating times.

STEPS TO A HEALTHY WEIGHT

For a moment, put aside thoughts of weight loss and dieting and looking thin — think about what it means to simply be healthy. The steps outlined in this book — particularly eating a healthy, plant-based diet with a moderate consumption of alcohol; moving and exercising; getting enough sleep; handling stress; and maximizing social support — are also the ones that will help you attain a healthy weight.

DIFFERENT STROKES

A population that's long been held up to promote diets high in animal fat is the Inuit, who live in Arctic areas. But here's the thing you don't often hear about: Around two-thirds of the Inuit have a genetic mutation that prevents their cholesterol from skyrocketing on this high animal fat, low-carb diet. The rest of the world's population just isn't built this way.

The key to a lifelong healthy weight isn't an over-restrictive diet, compulsive exercise or a particular combination of food. It's all of these healthy habits put together that will help you shed excess pounds, enjoy a more active, energetic life and reduce your risk of many diseases.

Eating a healthy diet

Studies have shown that a variety of healthy eating patterns can help you lose weight. Advocates of low-fat and low-carb diets, the Mediterranean diet, intermittent energy restriction and fasting diets all can point to studies that show these diets have produced weight loss, although the evidence is mostly for short-term weight loss.

But all too often, "going on a diet" also involves "getting off" at some point. And in many cases, the weight that's lost initially is eventually regained. So the best "diet" is the one you can stick with for the long term.

I'm a fan of the Mediterranean diet because it's a prescription for a lifelong pattern of healthy eating, rather than a strict set of rules that are hard to follow. And the Mediterranean pattern of eating has been shown to reduce your risk of serious chronic illnesses like heart disease, diabetes, cancer and dementia. Chapter 8 discusses the Mediterranean diet in detail.

If you eat more vegetables, fruits, whole grains, lean protein and low-fat dairy; a handful of nuts; and olive oil as your main source of fat, you're likely eating less high-calorie, energy-dense foods — foods like doughnuts, sugary breakfast cereals, steak, bacon, butter, heavy sauces, ice cream and especially ultraprocessed foods. In fact, eating a healthy vegetarian diet is likely the best way to promote coronary artery disease regression and weight loss.

Whether you follow a vegetarian diet or not, replacing high-calorie foods with low-calorie foods reduces the total number of calories you're taking in, even if you're still eating the same volume of food. Over time, this reduction in calories will lead to weight loss.

Traditionally, the Mediterranean diet has also included a small amount of red wine, generally with a meal. And studies have shown that red wine may have a slightly protective effect on heart health. If you drink alcohol, keep in mind that it's not calorie-free. Moderating your consumption of alcohol can help you take in fewer calories. Save wine for your meal or drinks for special occasions. Replace the wine in your wine glass with sparkling water every so often.

To be successful, make small changes slowly. And, as we discussed in Chapter 4, link each small change to something you already do. Cook with olive oil instead of butter. Or use just a small pat of butter to enhance the flavor of your food. At mealtime substitute one bite of a food that increases inflammation, such as meat, with a bite of vegetables from your plate.

Make changes that are so small they're easy to accomplish and you feel good about them. Since we all eat meals at least two or three times a day, making a small mealtime change over months to years can help us age slower and live longer, or live younger longer.

Keep in mind that the messages we're getting from the food industry might not match these common sense goals. For example, the mouth-watering ads we see for processed foods heavily outnumber the ads for fruits and vegetables.

Why is that? It may not completely explain it, but the profit margin for sales of processed foods approaches 90%, while it's only 10% for fruits and vegetables. The odds are clearly stacked against us when it comes to healthy eating.

Moving and exercising

Losing weight, at least initially, is almost completely about eating fewer calories. But most people get to a point where their weight loss levels off. That's when a little bit of physical activity can go a long way.

If you only cut calories to lose weight — without increasing your physical activity — you lose muscle. Muscle loss makes it harder to keep weight off because muscle tissue burns calories, even at rest.

In Chapter 9, we talk about high intensity interval training and how even doing just three intervals of exercise 10 minutes at a time can help when you hit your weight-loss plateau.

As with healthy eating patterns, the best form of exercise is the kind that you enjoy and will want to do regularly. You don't have to start running marathons (although you can if you want). Start small, maybe doing a pushup or two during commercial breaks on your favorite TV show or after brushing your teeth, or doing a short bit of yoga before bed. Whenever you can, make an excuse to be more active, not less.

Getting enough sleep

You may have heard that getting too little sleep can lead to weight gain. Is this true? It may be. Although the evidence isn't conclusive, some studies suggest that consistently sleeping less than five hours — or more than nine hours — a night increases the likelihood of weight gain.

In one study, sleep deprivation in men increased their calorie intake the next day. In another study, women who slept less than five hours or more than nine hours a night were more likely to gain weight over five to seven years compared with women who slept seven hours a night. A more recent study of middle-aged women found an association between short sleep duration and being overweight.

One explanation for the connection may be that sleep duration affects hormones regulating hunger — ghrelin and leptin — and stimulates the appetite. Other contributing factors may be that lack of sleep leads to fatigue and results in less physical activity or that longer awake hours lead to more eating. It's also possible that factors linked to both weight and sleep, such as sleep apnea or high blood pressure, may confound the relationship between the two.

Getting a good night's sleep is important for many reasons. It can make you feel more rested, alert and motivated to perform daily tasks and meet unexpected challenges. A better mood helps you feel more in control of your day and better able to make healthy choices, including eating well and exercising. An added bonus of sleeping well may very well be maintaining a healthy weight.

Stress and weight gain

When you're under stress, it can be harder to eat healthy. For example, you might think, I'm already under so much stress, I can't possibly be expected to choose this salad over that cheesy pizza. Also, during times of particularly high stress, we tend to use food as a way to fulfill emotional needs — sometimes called stress eating or emotional eating. And we may be especially likely to eat high-calorie foods during times of stress, even when we're not hungry. After a hard day, for example, the only way we can think of to relax is with a big bowl of buttered popcorn or ice cream.

Managing stress can help us prevent weight gain from this kind of overeating and reduce the risk of obesity. When we feel less stressed and more in control of our lives, it's easier to stick to healthy eating and exercise habits.

Everyone handles stress differently. But notice if you tend to cope with stress by eating. Even small amounts add up. Going from a BMI of 25 to a BMI of 30 over a period of three decades requires only an extra 10 calories a day. It's not unlike compound interest — the reason that your savings account can slowly grow over time to become quite large. Albert Einstein called compound interest one of the most powerful forces in the universe!

Try these stress management techniques to combat stress-related weight gain:
- Have a plan in place for a de-stressing activity that doesn't involve food. It could be something simple like watching the birds in your birdfeeder or listening to relaxing background music in your office. Make sure it's an activity you enjoy.
- If you do find yourself contemplating food when you're stressed out, ask yourself why you're eating — are you truly hungry or do you feel stressed or anxious?
- If you're tempted to eat when you're not hungry, find a distraction. Or have some low-calorie food options ready to go such as carrots, broccoli or cucumber sticks dipped in a yogurt-based dressing.
- Don't skip the basics of stress management: Engage in regular physical activity or exercise, get adequate sleep, and seek encouragement from friends and family.

'FAT BUT FIT'

Some scientists have found that it may be possible to be "fat but fit." In a 2016 study involving almost 30,000 men and women, researchers looked into the relationship between BMI, aerobic (cardiorespiratory) fitness and mortality. Study participants were divided up by whether they fell below or above a body mass index (BMI) of 30 and by how fit they were. Fitness was measured by how well participants did on an exercise test — how many metabolic equivalents (METs) they could attain. METs indicate how much oxygen your tissues receive and use during exercise. For example, one MET is the energy required to sit quietly. The higher the MET reading you can achieve on a treadmill exercise test, the better shape you're in.

Predictably, the group considered the healthiest included those with a BMI under 30 and able to go over 10 METs. But the next healthiest group included those with a BMI over 30 who were also able to go over 10 METs. The group most likely to shorten their life spans? Those who had a BMI under 30 but couldn't hit at least 10 METs — not obese but also not fit. The moral of the exercise story: Fitness improves your health, regardless of how much you weigh. And ignoring fitness threatens your health.

The concept of "fat but fit" probably comes as a surprise to many because we've been trained to think that thin equals healthy. But here's one possible explanation for the study findings: When you become fit you lose a lot of that troublesome excess abdominal fat. Abdominal fat releases chemicals into the bloodstream that are proinflammatory, which increases your risk of diseases such as heart disease, cancer and Alzheimer's disease.

Maximizing support

All of the healthy habits listed above are much easier to maintain when we have the support of family and friends. It's true that only you can decide how you will live. But having the emotional and practical support of others can make your healthy decisions a lot more enjoyable — and sustainable.

Plus, the decision to adopt healthier habits isn't a one-time decision — it's a daily, and sometimes hourly, recommitment. There will be times when we need some extra strength.

Some members of your support team will be the people closest to you, such as your spouse or best friend. Others might come from unexpected corners of your life — a co-worker who's striving to be more active or a long-distance relative with whom you can swap instant messages about your latest successes. And studies have shown that supporting others not only helps them, it helps you feel better about yourself.

A PRODUCT OF OUR HABITS

What we weigh when we step on a scale is in large part a product of our long-term habits. Temporary diets may help us lose a few pounds but these diets are generally unsustainable.

Just as our daily choices can lead us to gain weight over time, so too can our choices help us undo that gain. We probably won't be able to undo it all at once. But if each day we choose to turn ever so slightly toward a

THE HALO EFFECT OF A HEALTHY HABIT

If you view exercise as more of an opportunity for sociaiizing rather than an intense solo workout, you might have a leg up on longevity. Results from a large study out of Denmark show that social sports are linked to lower mortality than individual, or nonsocial, sports. Sports that require two or more participants — in this study, tennis, badminton and soccer — appear to be associated with the best improvements in longevity. This is even though the people who play social sports tend to engage in less total active time a week than those involved in individual sports, such as cycling or working out at a gym.

The Denmark study was observational in nature, so it can't prove definitively that social sports add years to a person's life. But the association was pretty strong, probably for multiple reasons. The first reason is that you're more likely to actually do the sport when you're part of a team or when teammates are waiting for you to show up to play. Also, interacting with others and being part of a group may provide added benefits such as stress reduction and camaraderie. Indeed, other studies show that social support is a very strong protector of health, even more so than not smoking, staying lean or having a normal blood pressure.

healthier long-term eating plan — one less bite of burger here, one more of vegetables there — we will gradually build up to a healthy, sustainable eating pattern. No change is too small or too late.

And don't forget the other steps, which all do their own part in contributing toward a healthy weight and a healthy life — find ways to be active and fit that make you happy, prioritize quality sleep time, make it a point to relax and connect with others, avoid pollutants and toxins such as smoking and vaping, and enjoy alcohol in moderation (if at all). Life gets complicated, no doubt, as I know all too well. But I also know that going back to these simple basics will help me and you live younger longer. Cheers!

Having healthy habits in one area, such as exercise, tends to lead to better health in other areas of life, such as social support. And vice versa. I call this the "halo effect." The halo surrounding exercising with friends radiates additional health effects such as more activity and social support, less stress, better blood pressure, lower cholesterol, and lower weight.

Life expectancy increases with social sports

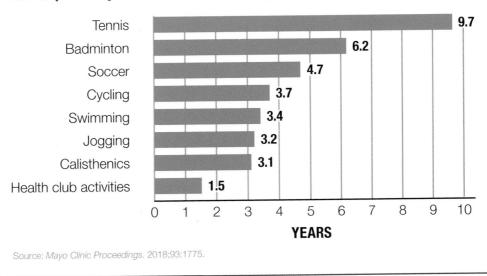

Source: *Mayo Clinic Proceedings*. 2018;93:1775.

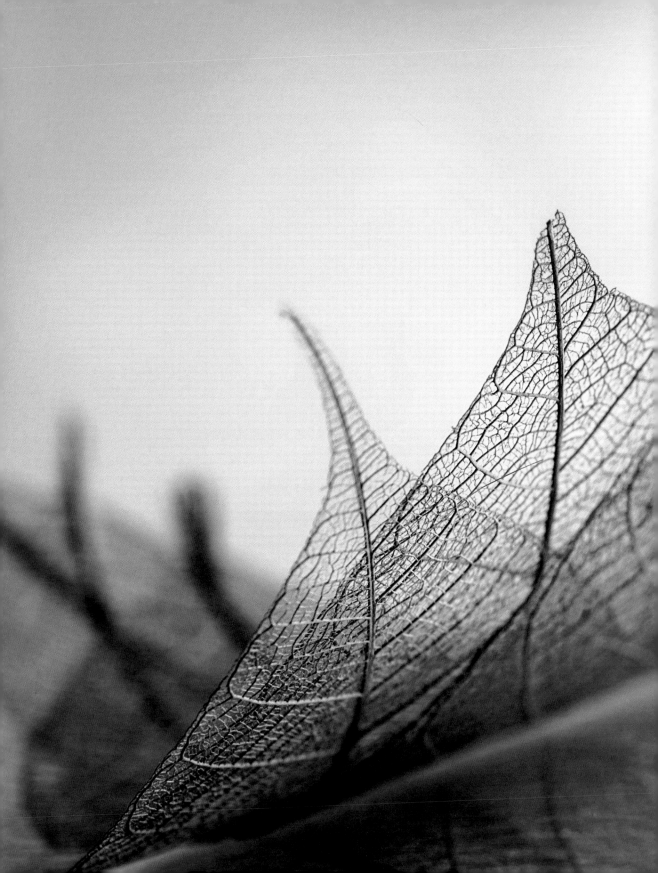

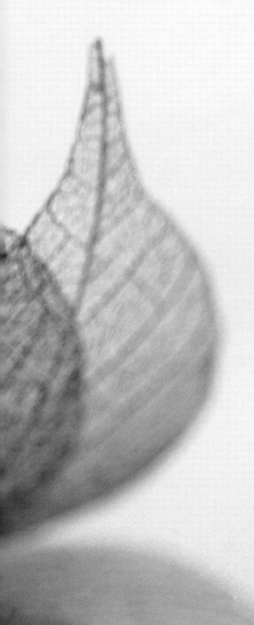

PART 3

Additional help

GATHER YOUR TOOLS

To do some of the physical assessments in this section, you'll need:

- ☐ A stopwatch or a watch that can measure seconds

- ☐ A flexible tape measure

- ☐ A scale

- ☐ Someone to help you record your scores and count repetitions

You'll also need a pencil or pen and paper to record your scores as you complete an assessment. You can record your scores in a notebook or journal, or save them in a spreadsheet or another electronic format.

Assessments, tips and resources

To know where you're going on your health journey, it helps to have a baseline. This part of the book includes a variety of assessments, tips and resources to help you evaluate where you are in maintaining your overall health.

Some of the physical self-assessments involve movement and moderately intense exercise. If you don't have any health concerns and you're in fairly good physical condition, go ahead and get started. If you have health issues — conditions such as cardiovascular disease, high blood pressure or respiratory disease — or you have concerns about your health, talk to your doctor or health care provider first to make sure it's safe for you to perform the activities.

Also, don't view these assessments as a substitute for seeing your doctor. Regular evaluations are important because there are some health conditions — your blood cholesterol, blood sugar levels and the health of your bones, for example — that you can't detect on your own with a self-assessment.

WHAT'S YOUR BMI?

To determine your body mass index (BMI), find your height in the left column. Follow that row across to the weight nearest yours. Look at the top of that column for your approximate BMI.

BMI	Normal		Overweight					Obese				
	19	24	25	26	27	28	29	30	35	40	45	50
Height	Weight in pounds											
4'10"	91	115	119	124	129	134	138	143	167	191	215	239
4'11"	94	119	124	128	133	138	143	148	173	198	222	247
5'0"	97	123	128	133	138	143	148	153	179	204	230	255
5'1"	100	127	132	137	143	148	153	158	185	211	238	264
5'2"	104	131	136	142	147	153	158	164	191	218	246	273
5'3"	107	135	141	146	152	158	163	169	197	225	254	282
5'4"	110	140	145	151	157	163	169	174	204	232	262	291
5'5"	114	144	150	156	162	168	174	180	210	240	270	300
5'6"	118	148	155	161	167	173	179	186	216	247	278	309
5'7"	121	153	159	166	172	178	185	191	223	255	287	319
5'8"	125	158	164	171	177	184	190	197	230	262	295	328
5'9"	128	162	169	176	182	189	196	203	236	270	304	338
5'10"	132	167	174	181	188	195	202	209	243	278	313	348
5'11"	136	172	179	186	193	200	208	215	250	286	322	358
6'0"	140	177	184	191	199	206	213	221	258	294	331	368
6'1"	144	182	189	197	204	212	219	227	265	302	340	378
6'2"	148	186	194	202	210	218	225	233	272	311	350	389
6'3"	152	192	200	208	216	224	232	240	279	319	359	399
6'4"	156	197	205	213	221	230	238	246	287	328	369	410

Source: National Institutes of Health, 1998.

WAIST MEASUREMENT

Finding out your waist measurement can help you gauge your risk of health problems. Locate the highest point on each hipbone and, using a flexlble tape measure, measure horizontally around your abdomen just above these points.

Category	BMI	Waist circumference	
		Men: 40" or less Women: 35" or less	Men: Over 40" Women: Over 35"
Normal	18.5-24.9		
Overweight	25-29.9	Increased risk	High risk
Obese	30-34.9 35-39.9	High risk Very high risk	Very high risk Very high risk
Extreme obesity	40 or over	Extremely high risk	Extremely high risk

Source: Circulation. 2014;129(suppl 2):S102.

WAIST-TO-HIP RATIO

To obtain your hip circumference, measure at the fullest part of your hips. Don't pull the measuring tape tightly against your skin.

Calculate your waist-to-hip ratio by dividing your waist circumference by your hip circumference. Don't hold your belly in while measuring.

Waist-to-hip ratio	Men	Women
Healthy	0.9 or less	0.85 or less
Increased risk of heart disease	1.0 or more	1.0 or more

Source: World Health Organization

CARDIOVASCULAR FITNESS

The best method to test cardiovascular fitness is called a maximal oxygen consumption test, which is usually performed on a treadmill in a doctor's office or a hospital. It's a test adults over 40 should have done.

If you're in relatively good health, you can estimate your cardiovascular fitness at home using the 1.5-mile walk/run test. This test approximates your fitness level

ESTIMATED FITNESS LEVEL BASED ON 1.5-MILE WALK/RUN*

Fitness level	Age					
	20-29	30-39	40-49	50-59	60-69	70+
Men	Time to complete 1.5 miles (minutes and seconds)					
Superior to excellent		10:47-8:49	11:16-9:10	12:07-9:34	13:23-10:09	14:34-10:28
Fair to good	12:28-10:45	13:04-11:06	13:49-11:41	15:03-12:36	16:46-13:53	18:38-15:13
Very poor to poor	21:25-12:53	20:58-13:24	22:20-14:07	25:01-15:20	26:18-17:11	32:45-19:30
Women	Time to complete 1.5 miles (minutes and seconds)					
Superior to excellent	11:58-9:29	12:25-9:51	13:22-10:09	14:34-11:22	16:21-11:58	17:38-11:58
Fair to good	14:50-12:25	15:38-12:53	16:21-13:32	18:07-15:11	20:06-16:46	21:34-18:14
Very poor to poor	23:58-15:14	24:47-15:58	25:49-16:46	28:39-18:37	30:13-20:46	36:12-22:20

*Norms based on Cooper Clinic patients.

Source: *Physical Fitness Assessments and Norms for Adults and Law Enforcement.* The Cooper Institute; 2013.

based on how quickly you're able to traverse 1.5 miles. Wear comfortable clothing and sturdy walking or running shoes. Walk on a flat surface, such as a standard quarter-mile track (six laps equal 1.5 miles) or a flat road where you've measured the distance of 1.5 miles with your car's odometer. Use a stopwatch or a watch with a second hand to record your time.

Warm up by walking slowly for three to five minutes. When you're ready to begin, start the clock and begin walking or running as fast as you can while maintaining a steady pace. You can slow down and speed up as you wish, but the goal is to complete the 1.5 miles as quickly as possible. When finished, keep walking for a few minutes to cool down and follow up with a few stretches.

Compare your results to the table nearby according to your age and sex. While the test is fairly easy to do on your own, it isn't perfect. But it can provide a baseline assessment of your cardiovascular health that you can improve on.

⚠ EXERCISE CAUTIONS

Don't attempt this test if you have a heart condition, lung disease or other chronic illness, or you haven't been routinely walking for 15 to 20 minutes several times a week. Talk to your doctor about how to assess your current fitness level and how best to improve it. Also, don't perform this test on a treadmill because a treadmill will skew your results.

Stop exercising and rest if you have:
- Tightness, pressure or pain in your chest.
- Pain in your arm, shoulder, neck or jaw.
- Severe shortness of breath.
- Lightheadedness, dizziness or confusion.
- Stomach pain.
- Nausea, vomiting or headache.
- Extreme or unusual fatigue.

Tell your doctor or health care provider if you experience any of these.

PUSHUP TEST

A common way to assess muscular strength and endurance is to see how many pushups you can do without losing good form. If you haven't been very active lately, do modified pushups on your knees. If you're generally fit and able to do classic full-body pushups, do those.

Compare your results with the chart below. Even if you fall into one of the lower categories, keep in mind that you can always improve your fitness. Start with one pushup a day; no need to make it a long, drawn-out procedure. Then just see how many you can do.

PUSHUP TEST RESULTS

Fitness level	Age				
	20-29	30-39	40-49	50-59	60+
Men	**Number of full-body pushups**				
Superior to Excellent	47-100	39-86	30-64	25-51	23-39
Fair to good	29-44	24-36	18-29	13-24	10-22
Very poor to poor	13-27	9-24	5-16	3-11	2-9
Women	**Number of full-body pushups**				
Superior to Excellent	36-70	31-56	24-60	21-31	15-20
Fair to good	23-34	19-29	13-21	12-20	5-15
Very poor to poor	9-15	4-17	1-11	0-10	0-4

*Norms based on worksite wellness program participants at Texas Instruments.

Source: *Physical Fitness Assessments and Norms for Adults and Law Enforcement.* The Cooper Institute; 2013.

BASIC STRETCHING EXERCISES

It's important to give your body time to adjust both before and after an exercise session. The following stretches can help you warm up your muscles and gradually increase your heart rate, breathing and blood flow before you exercise. After you exercise, the same stretches can help your body cool down.

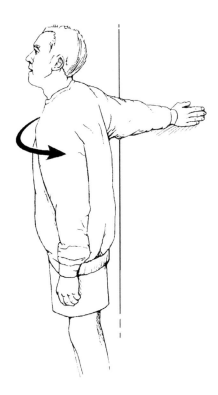

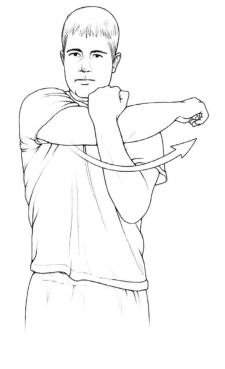

▶ CHEST STRETCH

1. Stand next to a wall. Extend your right arm and place your outstretched palm against the wall.
2. Turn your body away from your arm until you feel the stretch.
3. Repeat with your left arm.

▶ SHOULDER STRETCH

1. Lift your left arm to the level of your chest.
2. Place your right hand on your left elbow and gently pull your left arm across your chest.
3. Repeat with your right arm.

Do the stretches slowly and gently. Stretch to the point that you feel a definite pulling sensation in the muscle but not to the point of pain. Hold each position for 30 seconds. Relax and breathe normally.

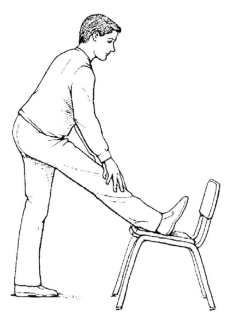

▶ HAMSTRING STRETCH

1. Stand and rest one leg on a chair or bench directly in front of you. If your balance is poor, hang on to something for stability.
2. Lean forward until you feel a stretch in the back of your thigh.
3. Repeat using your other leg.

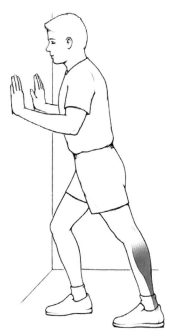

▶ CALF STRETCH

1. Place your palms on a wall and stand an arm's length away from it.
2. Bring one leg forward and bend that knee while keeping the opposite leg straight and your heel on the floor.
3. Lean forward until you feel a stretch in the back of the opposite leg.
4. Never bend your knee so it goes past your toe. If you need to intensify this stretch, move your extended leg farther back.
5. Repeat with the other leg.

If you occasionally have to shorten your stretching time, begin your preferred activity at a slow pace and then gradually increase your pace. Be sure to stretch well during your cool-down.

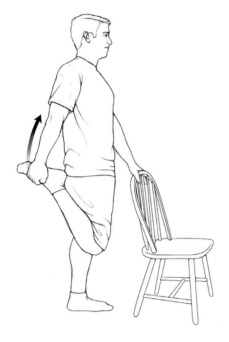

▶ QUADRICEPS AND HIP FLEXOR STRETCH

1. Stand and place your left hand on a wall or a sturdy piece of furniture to help you balance.
2. Grasp your right foot or ankle with your right hand. Tighten your abdominal muscles.
3. Slowly pull your right leg back until you feel a stretch in the front of your right thigh and hip. Do not bend forward. Keep knees together.
4. Repeat using your left leg.

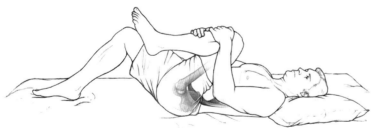

▶ LOWER BACK STRETCH (KNEE TO CHEST)

1. Lie on your back on a firm surface with your hips and knees bent and feet flat.
2. Pull your left knee toward your left shoulder by placing your hands on your knee. Pull gently until you feel a stretch in your lower back.
3. Repeat with your right knee (keeping your left foot flat).
4. Finally, bring both knees toward your shoulders.

DIET INVENTORY

How do you eat now? Take an inventory of your current eating pattern using the chart below. If you answer yes to a question, put a 1 next to that question. Then add up your total points. To be on the healthy side, your goal should be 11 or more points.

Do you use olive oil as your main cooking fat?

Do you use an olive oil-based sauce at least twice a week?

Do you consume 4 tablespoons or more a day of olive oil?

Do you eat four or more servings a day of vegetables? *One serving is one cup raw veggies or ½ cup cooked veggies.*

Do you eat three or more servings a day of fruit? *One serving is one whole medium-sized fruit or about 1 cup of fresh fruit.*

Do you eat three or more servings a week of beans, such as kidney or black beans, or legumes, such as split peas or lentils? *One serving is ½ cup cooked beans.*

Do you eat four or more servings a week of nuts? *One serving is ¼ cup.*

Do you eat three or more servings a week of fish or shellfish? *One serving is 3 to 5 ounces of fish or 6 to 7 ounces of shellfish.*

Do you usually eat chicken or turkey (white meat, no skin)?

Do you eat one serving or less a day of meat, such as hamburger, beef, veal, lamb, venison, pork, ham or sausage? *One serving is 3 ounces.*

Do you eat one serving or less a day of butter, margarine or cream? *One serving is 1 teaspoon.*

Do you drink one can or less a day of carbonated cola? *One can is 12 ounces.*

Do you eat three servings or less a week of sweets or pastries, such as cake, cookies, biscuits or custard?

Do you drink one glass of wine a day? *One glass is equal to 5 ounces for men and 3 ounces for women. Do not add more points if you drink more wine than this. Do not add points for any other kind of alcohol you may drink.*

Total score

WHAT'S A SINGLE SERVING?

	Calories	Visual cue
Vegetables		
1 cup cut-up vegetables	25	1 baseball
2 cups raw, leafy greens	25	2 baseballs
Fruits		
½ cup sliced fruit	60	1 tennis ball
1 small apple or medium orange	60	1 tennis ball
Carbohydrates		
½ cup plain pasta or dried cereal	70	Hockey puck
½ small whole-grain bagel	70	Hockey puck
1 slice whole-grain bread	70	Hockey puck
½ medium plain baked potato	70	Hockey puck
Protein/Dairy		
3 ounces fish	110	Deck of cards
2-2½ ounces chicken	110	Deck of cards
1½ ounces lean beef	110	½ deck of cards
1½-2 ounces low-fat hard cheese	110	⅓ deck of cards
Fats		
1½ teaspoons peanut butter	45	2 dice
1 teaspoon butter or margarine	45	1 die

ASSESS YOUR PRIORITIES

Assessing your priorities can help you manage stress. Use the quadrant below to help you map out areas in your life to prioritize and areas to let go of.

Place factors in your life that are very important to you toward the top. Place factors that aren't that important toward the bottom. You can further qualify these factors by the amount of control you have over them (less control toward the left, more control toward the right). There are some examples already there to help you get started.

When you've finished, take a look at the upper right quadrant. These are the factors that are important to you that you can control. Brainstorm ways you can focus your energy more on these factors while reducing the time and energy spent on less important factors, particularly those you can't control.

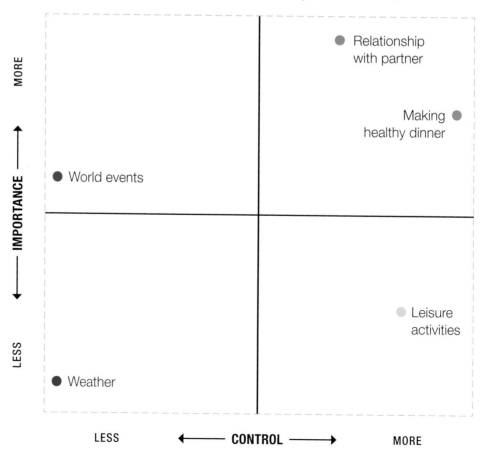

EVALUATE YOUR STRESS RESPONSE

Many people fall into the habit of making unhealthy choices when faced with stress. How you respond to a stressor is your choice. With planning and practice, you can control your responses to stressful situations. Consider the following unhealthy and healthy responses.

Unhealthy responses	Healthy responses
Angry outbursts	Taking time for exercise
Increased use of alcohol, tobacco, or drugs	Using relaxation techniques
Increased eating or shopping	Getting adequate sleep
Neglecting responsibilities	Learning to prioritize
Excessive worrying	Setting realistic goals
Procrastinating	Caring for yourself first

▶ CHECKLIST: TAKE CONTROL

☐ Identify healthy strategies for dealing with stressors you can control.

☐ Change your view of a stressor that is beyond your control.

☐ Focus on self-care (exercise regularly, eat well, connect to support systems, take time for pleasurable activities).

☐ Practice relaxation techniques and other positive habits such as time management, anger management, positive self-talk and realistic thinking.

☐ Know when to "let go."

Other resources

American Heart Association
www.heart.org

Centers for Disease Control and Prevention
www.cdc.gov

Mayo Clinic
www.MayoClinic.org

Mayo Clinic Connect
https://connect.MayoClinic.org
Online community where you can connect with others like you, ask questions and share your experience

Mayo Clinic's YouTube channel
www.youtube.com/user/MayoClinic
Keyword search: Kopecky

Oldways: Cultural food traditions
https://oldwayspt.org

Heart Risk Calculator
www.cvriskcalculator.com
Based on 2013 American Heart Association Guideline on the Assessment of Cardiovascular Risk

ASCVD Risk Estimator Plus
www.tools.acc.org/ASCVD-Risk-Estimator-Plus or download the app

Selected recommended reading

Atomic Habits
by James Clear. Avery; 2018.

Good Habits, Bad Habits:
The Science of Making
Positive Changes That Stick
by Wendy Wood. Farrar, Straus and
Giroux; 2019.

Mini Habits: Smaller Habits,
Bigger Results
by Stephen Guise. CreateSpace; 2013.

Tiny Habits: The Small Changes
That Change Everything
by BJ Fogg, Ph.D. Mariner Books; 2021.

The Mayo Clinic Guide to
Stress-Free Living
by Amit Sood, M.D. Da Capo
Lifelong Books; 2013.

The Power of Habit: Why We Do
What We Do in Life and Business
by Charles Duhigg. Random House;
2012.

The One-Minute Workout:
Science Shows a Way To Get Fit
That's Smarter, Faster, Shorter
by Martin Gibala, Ph.D. Avery; 2017.

Index

Page references in italics indicate illustrations, and t *indicates a table.*

genetic mutations linked to, 24
health span shortened by, 37
heart age and, 20, *21*
as leading cause of death, 15–16, 72, 95
among millennials, 60
oxygen consumption stress test and, 121–22
risk factors for, 20, 25, 39
sleep's effects on, 135, *138–39*
smoking as causing, 167

heart risk calculator, 212

high blood pressure
alcohol-related, 179
diet and, 96
lowering, 130
among millennials, 60
quality of life diminished by, 19
sleep's effects on, 135

HIIT (high-intensity interval training), 122, 124–31, *129*

homeostasis, 24, 136

HPA (hypothalamic-pituitary-adrenal) axis, 148

Huntington's disease, 24

I

immune system, 83–91
adaptive, 86, *87*
COVID-19 and, 83–86, *85*, *87*, 89, 91
exercise and, 88–89
heavy drinking as weakening, 181
inflammation following immune response, 86
innate, 86
mask wearing and, 84
nutrition and, 87–89
sleep and, 88, 134–35
stress and, 88–91, 149
See also inflammation

infectious diseases, 15–16
See also specific diseases

inflammation
acid reflux, 29–30, 168
body fat linked with, 118
chronic, 27, *27–28*, 29–33, *30*, 88–89
coronary artery disease caused by, 29
diet and, 27, 28, 32, 98–99
exercise/physical activity and, 32, 118
following immune response, 86
nature/being outdoors and, 153
sleep and, 91, 135
from smoking, 166
stress and, 27, 29, 33

influenza, 15–16, 86

insomnia, 142

insulin, 37, 118–19, 130–31, 135, *137*, 150–51

intermittent fasting, 189

Inuit people, 189

K

Kennedy, John F., 164

ketosis, 189

L

Lancet diet study, 95, 110

leukocytes, 27

life expectancy, 37

life span, average, 35, *36*, 37

lifestyle changes, 43–55
big results from small changes, 44–45
during COVID-19 pandemic, 84
failure and, *45*, 46
motivation and, 47, 49, 52
vs. sudden, drastic changes, 43–44
willpower and, 43, 46, 55
See also habits

Y